COMMUNICATION *and* EDUCATION SKILLS:
The Dietitian's Guide

COMMUNICATION *and* EDUCATION SKILLS: *The Dietitian's Guide*

BETSY B. HOLLI, Ed.D., R.D.

Associate Professor
Department of Home Economics
Rosary College
River Forest, Illinois

RICHARD J. CALABRESE, Ph.D.

Chairperson
Department of Communication
Arts and Sciences
Rosary College
River Forest, Illinois

Lea & Febiger   *Philadelphia*

Lea & Febiger
600 Washington Square
Philadelphia, PA   19106-4198
U.S.A.
(215) 922-1330

Library of Congress Cataloging-in-Publication Data

Holli, Betsy B.
    Communication and education skills.

    Includes index.
        1. Communication in diet therapy.   2. Patient
education.   3. Interpersonal communication.
I. Calabrese, Richard J.   II. Title.   [DNLM:
1. Communication.   2. Dietetics—education.
3. Interpersonal Relations.   WB 18 H739c]
RM214.3.H65   1986   613.2   86-10576
ISBN 0-8121-0974-0

PRINTED IN THE UNITED STATES OF AMERICA

Print No.   4   3   2

To Melvin G. Holli

and

To my mother, father, and mother-in-law—Vic and Jean Calabrese, and Jo Jaske—and to my wife, Alice Calabrese, for loving and tolerating me during this past year, during most of which I have been habitually and compulsively preoccupied.

FOREWORD

Today's dietetic educators and practitioners recognize the need for future dietitians to be not only knowledgeable in interpersonal skills, but also proficient in the use of such skills. Every practicing dietitian desires to be successful in his relationships with patients, clients, personnel, colleagues, and other professionals. Regardless of the emphasis of practice, whether administrative or clinical, dietitians are agents of change. To be effective in this role, they must be competent in applying the "helping skills" to bring about desirable changes in the behaviors of clients and/or personnel.

Drs. Holli and Calabrese respond to this need by bringing together in one book a substantive discussion of the major skills usually identified as contributing toward positive and harmonious human relationships. Traditionally, dietetic students have acquired knowledge of these skills through several of their courses, but have received little assistance in transferring the knowledge to practice. This book overcomes this deficiency by providing examples that apply each skill to multiple areas of dietetic practice. Suggested activities are included to reinforce the concepts presented.

Clearly, the need for communication skills is not bound by specialty area of practice or by profession. Therefore, the book will be useful to all health care providers as a regular reference for improving and maintaining their "helping skills." Students should be encouraged to use this text as a ready reference in their future daily practice.

Betty L. Beach, Ph.D., R.D.
Director, Dietetic Internship
Edward Hines, Jr. Hospital—Veterans Administration

PREFACE

The purpose of this book is to introduce and review the major communication and education skills that dietitians and nutritionists use in professional practice. The idea for the book grew from a perceived need for a publication dealing with these skills. A large number of publications cover the technical knowledge, skills, and expertise needed by dietitians, but ignore the human skills required of the health care professional in working with others. One's professional goals cannot be realized without learning interpersonal skills; one must be able to establish and maintain an effective relationship with the person needing one's knowledge and skills. Today's dietitians need to enlarge their roles and abilities as communicators, interviewers, counselors, educators, trainers, information interpreters, facilitative problem-solvers, motivators, and behavioral change specialists.

The development of skills in communication and education is not an end in itself, but rather the basis for effective relationships with others. Health professionals engage in both verbal and nonverbal communication with patients and clients in interviewing, counseling, and educating them. The quality of this communication can determine the degree to which the intervention benefits the individual. Dietitians in administrative positions discover that communication skills are essential to leadership and managerial effectiveness, and that they produce the greatest return from human resources. In addition to developing functional one-on-one relationships, dietitians must be able to work with groups.

Our book introduces the communication and education principles, techniques, and intervention strategies available to dietitians interacting with clients, patients, employees, and others. A variety of methods is presented, since there is no one best way to communicate. There are a number of strategies for nutritional counseling, for example, and the practitioner has to determine which ones best fit his style, and which are likely to be most effective with specific individuals. Knowing a variety of communication skills prepares the dietitian to work with clients on a contingency basis.

Communication skills can be learned only through practice. Through frequent attempts to improve and hone his skills, the dietitian will notice a difference in the way others respond, both personally and professionally. The text is interspersed with examples for clarification, and following each chapter is a selection of exercises. We encourage readers to experiment with one or two skills daily, especially those with which they are unfamiliar. The skills can be practiced on family, friends, and colleagues, and incorporated into one's practice. For the beginner, the book need not be read cover to cover. The optimal time for studying the material is when one is in a position to use it.

In selecting the content for the book, we examined the American Dietetic Association's role delineation studies, which describe the major and specific responsibilities, requisite knowledge, and skills needed for the practice of clinical dietetics, community dietetics, and food service systems management. In addition, we reviewed the literature of dietetics, solicited the opinions of practitioners, and spent time working with dietitians in various areas of practice. During the preparation of the manuscript, we were encouraged by the publication of the Report of the 1984 Study Commission on Dietetics, which recommends a greater emphasis on communication.

Entire books are written on the subjects of most of the chapters and even on some subjects within the chapters. Although every topic could not be treated in detail, we hope that the book will stimulate further interest and exploration.

While the book was written primarily for dietetic students and practitioners, the same basic skills are used by most health professionals and people in leadership roles. Since the dietitian is not the only person dealing with nutritional problems, the book may prove useful to others, such as health educators, public health nurses, dietetic technicians, dietary managers, and home economists.

While we are aware of the fact that dietitians are predominantly women, and health care recipients and employees are both men and women, we have used the traditional masculine pronouns throughout the book to avoid "he/she" and other cumbersome forms. The intended meaning includes women as well as men, and the terms "helper," "health professional," "communicator," "interviewer," "counselor," "trainer," "educator," and the like, are used when the dietitian assumes these roles and responsibilities.

We wish to thank Ann B. Williams, Ph.D., for contributing the important chapter on behavior modification. We are indebted to a number of registered dietitians and others who were helpful in providing judicious advice about the manuscript, in arranging for us to spend time in professional practice, or in sharing ideas as they were working and we were observing. These individuals include Doris Aird, Martha Atkins, Betty Beach, Diane Berry, Judy Beto, Mary Castellanos, Helen Chu, Rebecca Dowling, Suzanne Kordesh, Jan Kowall, Mary Lesniewski, Evelyn Morrison, Jane Oakes, Georgann Pardee, Karen Rezebek, Joann Schulte, Shahida Shaffie, Cindy

Sherwood, Belle Shim, Diane Sowa, and Carol Zuehsow. None, of course, bears responsibility for the judgments contained herein, which are solely those of the authors. We would like to express our deep appreciation to Rosary College for granting sabbatical leaves so that the manuscript could be completed. Dr. Melvin G. Holli provided counsel, assistance, and support from commencement of the idea to the completion of the project.

The following people assisted in providing computers, software, and tutoring in word processing: the staff of the Waubonsee Community College Library, John Blair, Michael Zink, John Govern, and Mary Arlowe. Without their assistance, the experience of writing this book would not have been as creative or exciting. Mary Parks and George B. Beranek assisted with research and compiling bibliographies.

Betsy B. Holli
River Forest, Illinois   *Richard J. Calabrese*

CONTENTS

5 BEHAVIOR MODIFICATION
Ann B. Williams, Ph.D.   81

6 GROUP PROCESS   103

7 PLANNING LEARNING   127

1

Communication and Education Skills for Dietitians

Dietitians are expected to have good communication skills.[1] The job responsibilities of clinical and community dietitians involve communicating with patients, clients, and other professionals to educate them about nutrition. Administrative dietitians and managers, who communicate with and train subordinate employees, discover that communication skills are an important key to leadership and managerial effectiveness. Communication is considered a supporting field for dietetics, and a strengthening of communication skills for dietitians at all levels is strongly recommended.[2]

In recent years, health professionals, including dietitians and nutritionists, have become more aware of the necessity of acquiring skills in interpersonal relations, since a number of their job responsibilities require frequent interaction with others, such as clients, patients, employees, colleagues, and other health professionals. In addition to having the requisite technical skills, the dietitian must be able to relate effectively to others. It is not enough to demonstrate competency in one's subject; such competency must be put to use. Human relationships are described as "the media through which technical skills are practiced."[3] Thus there is a need to focus on the process of delivering to others such dietetic services as nutritional intervention through interpersonal communication, counseling, and education. In addition, coordination of team efforts for patient care clearly requires communication and cooperation. Communication is a link connecting all health team members, including the patient.

The scope of dietetics is broad, with dietitians and nutritionists employed in a variety of positions and in a number of different settings. The majority are employed in health care facilities (acute care hospitals, medical centers, and nursing homes), but others work in commercial business and industry, school feeding, or community and public health nutrition programs, or they are self-employed in private practice. In a survey, dietitians reported engaging in a wide range of professional activities, including food service management (food purchasing and supervision of employees); the nutritional care of clients and patients, and the management of clinical nutrition services; commercial activities (marketing and sales); the education of dietetic students and other health care professionals; nutrition education of the public; and administrative activities (fiscal planning and public relations).[4]

The six most common roles for the dietitian are clinical dietitian, administrative/food service management dietitian, generalist, dietetics or nutrition educator, community or public health nutritionist, and consultant. Each of these roles may be divided further into subspecialty groups. Within the American Dietetic Association (ADA) are the following 23 special interest groups:

Public health nutritionists
Gerontological nutrition
Dietetics in developmental and psychiatric disorders
Community nutrition research
Research dietitians
Renal dietitians
Dietitians in pediatric practice
Diabetes care and education
Dietitians in critical care
Dietetics in physical medicine and rehabilitation
Sports and cardiovascular nutritionists
Dietitians in general clinical practice
Consulting nutritionists—private practice
Consultant dietitians in health care facilities
Dietitians in business and industry
ADA members with management responsibilities in health care
     delivery systems
School food service
College and university food service
Clinical nutrition management
Dietetic educators of practitioners
Nutritionists in nursing education
Nutrition education for the public
Dietitians in medical and dental education

All of these specialists use communication skills and education skills in daily practice.

The American Dietetic Association has focused on the knowledge base necessary for professional practice and defined the requisite skills and competencies needed by practitioners. Since 1973, the ADA has been assessing and defining, through role delineation studies, the meaning of competence in the field of dietetics at the entry or minimum level.[5] Information from role delineation studies, which identify the knowledge needed to practice dietetics, is helpful in the credentialing process, in the education of practitioners, and in the process of assurance of quality service and practice.

Role delineation studies have identified the job responsibilities of entry-level dietitians related to communication and education, and the skills and knowledge needed for practice. Clinical dietitians, for example, are expected to plan, organize, implement, and evaluate nutrition education for clients and patients, give classes to groups, counsel individuals concerning nutrition concepts and desired changes in eating habits, and educate health team members on nutrition-related topics. Communicating plans for nutritional care to individuals or families, as well as to health team members, with documentation in the medical record, is a major responsibility. The development of orientation and training programs for subordinate clinical dietetic personnel is another function.[6]

In community dietetics, responsibilities include providing nutrition education to groups and to individual clients for health promotion, health maintenance, and rehabilitation, and developing orientation and training programs for support personnel.[7] Public health nutritionists and graduate faculty ranked "communicating clearly" and "performing direct dietary counseling" as the top two abilities necessary for practice.[8] In foodservice systems management, the dietitian is expected to interview applicants for identified positions, to orient and train personnel, to counsel subordinates, and to provide educational programs (on-the-job training, inservice training, and continuing education) that meet the needs of employees.[9] The consultant is a dietitian in private practice who confers with nursing homes and other institutions to provide advice, instructions, or recommendations for obtaining organizational objectives.

For interaction with those being advised, effective communication skills are a high priority.[1] Teaching is a function of most dietitians.

Common knowledge and skills needed by all dietitians for interpersonal relations include principles of verbal and nonverbal communication, principles and techniques of interviewing and counseling, theories and strategies for behavior modification and motivation, principles of learning, teaching methods and techniques, and knowledge of working with groups. These skills are not innate, but they can be learned and improved with practice.

In addition to devoting ongoing attention to the development of communication skills to improve his relationship with staff and clients, the dietitian needs to be professionally active in a communication network, which consists of people talking to one another and sharing ideas, information, and resources. It is essential for the dietitian to have an ongoing dialogue with other professionals in his area of expertise. One way to participate in such a dialogue is for the dietitian to join a professional interest group of fellow practitioners who wish to form a network in their area of interest and/or practice. Although sharing information is the primary purpose of networking, the contacts that networks provide are invaluable.

HELPING OTHERS

Dietetics is a "helping" profession concerned primarily with providing services beneficial to individuals and society, and dedicated to improving the nutritional status of people. Helping professions have been described as process professions that "require doing something with knowledge," such as communicating, interpreting, and applying nutritional science to the language and lifestyles of people to benefit their health.[1] The helping approach may also be utilized in managing subordinate staff. The professional seeks to guide others in bringing about change.[10]

Helping is a process involving a conversation or series of conversations with another person. Whether in social work, nursing, or dietetics, the professional seeks to answer the question: "What is helpful?" A great deal of helping involves problem solving. Resolving the problem may entail arriving at a decision; developing knowledge, insights, or mutual understanding; setting goals for change; or venting feelings. The client or patient requires the assistance of the professional in overcoming and solving his problem when he is unable to do so alone. He may be incapable of problem resolution, owing to lack of information, knowledge, skill, motivation, or resources, or owing to emotional feelings, such as anxiety.

Helping offers the potential for growth and development, and for achieving the intended result, which is change.[11] Brammer asserts that helping another person is a "process of enabling that person to grow in the direction he chooses."[12] Thus the client, not the helper, determines whether he wants help at all, and if he does, makes decisions about his needs and selects the goals for his change or growth. Clients and patients should not be perceived as passive recipients of services, but as active participants in their treatment in the health care process. Ultimately, the client or patient is responsible for his nutrition and health. The acceptance of help is voluntary, and the aim of the professional is to make the person self-sufficient so that eventually he can function on his own, solving future problems alone. Doing something for another without his initiative and consent may be counterproductive.

Since helping is future-oriented, counseling of both clients and employees focuses on what can be done to improve performance; it does not dwell on the failures of the past.[11] When he emphasizes what is acceptable to and possible for the individual rather than the individual's failure to comply with recommendations, the helper avoids labeling people as "uncooperative," "unmotivated," or "uninterested."

Problem solving involves listening, communicating, and educating, and is fundamentally a learning experience for the individual.[10] The interaction between the helper and the individual is a goal-oriented process through which change occurs in the form of learning new information, knowledge, or skills; gaining new insights and perspectives; modifying feelings; changing behaviors; and developing new resources as decisions are made and problems resolved. Helping is more than the provision of information. Almost anyone can supply information, and one does not need a professional to provide it. The resolution of problems, however, and the personal discovery of the meaning of solutions for his life come from the helper's interaction with the individual.

The professional and his client should engage in problem solving together, as partners, joining forces and interacting in seeking solutions to ensure an effective learning experience. Providing pat answers and quick solutions that may be obvious to the dietitian does not help the person learn to solve his problems, and this approach should be avoided. Initially, the professional needs to learn about the person and his circumstances in order to assess the problem and to plan to provide effective help. Through engaging in the problem solving process and exploring alternatives with the guidance and encouragement of the professional, the client gains insight into his own situation, makes decisions, sets goals, learns to manage his own resources, and brings about the salutary and desired changes that problem resolution entails. Involving the individual in solving his own problems greatly increases self-motivation.

The helping process takes place in the relationship developed between the helper and the individual client, which is a key to the effectiveness of helping and problem solving. The professional strives to create an environment of respect and trust by arranging and maintaining conditions in which the individual perceives himself as accepted, warmly received, valued, and understood. If the individual feels inferior, dependent, unappreciated, misunderstood, or manipulated, distrust can result, and the individual resists assistance. Trust must be earned; without it, vital self-disclosure on the part of the patient may be limited.[10] Trust in this sense means "the expectation that self-disclosure will be treated with respect and that feedback from the other can be relied on."[3] Respect and trust can be conveyed by not labeling the individual's responses "right" or "wrong," by providing privacy, by showing concern and understanding through careful listening, and by providing nonjudgmental verbal and nonverbal responses, including when necessary, accurate paraphrasing of the meaning of the individual's comments and feelings.

Relationships begin and develop through communication, and the quality of communication influences the quality of the relationship. According to Henderson, the single most important element in interpersonal communication is "sender credibility—the attitude the receiver of a message has toward the sender's trustworthiness." [13] Credibility gaps may occur when the helper fails to project warmth, empathy, friendliness, and concern.

The relationship between the professional and client is probably easiest to establish when the client is similar to the professional in educational level and socioeconomic status. There may be a potential problem when the client is very different from the professional. For example, professionals must deal with clients who are aged, illiterate, uneducated, hearing-impaired, alcoholic, or disabled. Clients may be of various religious, cultural, and ethnic groups, or may be people from lower socioeconomic groups than that of the professional. They may be individuals with critical injuries resulting from automobile accidents or burns, or people with life-threatening diseases such as cancer. The professional may need to examine his own values and personal attitudes toward others in developing effective interpersonal relationships. This self-awareness provides some insurance against prejudice, or against judging others by one's personal values, and enables the professional to function out of concern and respect for those who are different.

A number of skills are needed by helping professionals. These include techniques of interviewing and counseling; ability to relate to groups, individuals, and communities; effectiveness in bringing about change; capacity for self-understanding; establishment of professional, interdisciplinary relationships; and knowledge of personality, group, and societal dynamics. [10] With these skills, the helper can assist others to assess all dimensions of a problem, to explore alternative solutions, and to stimulate action toward positive change and problem resolution. The helper's proficiency in specific communication and helping skills directly affects the success or failure of helping transactions. Since considerable responsibility for desired outcomes must be assumed by the health professional, it is imperative that helpers develop and improve their counseling skills. [11]

PROMOTING CHANGE

The solutions discovered through the problem-solving process, whether used with clients or employees, require some kind of change from people. The client who is learning dietary changes, for example, may be expected to know and remember lists of foods that can or cannot be consumed, to read labels, to shop for and prepare different foods, or to use different cooking methods. An employee may need to learn and to follow new work methods and procedures.

Peck viewed the successful professional as a "change agent" who needed the ability to intervene in human environments to promote change in behavior. [14] Knowledge of the social, cultural, psychological, and other forces affecting motivation for change in individuals or in groups, either positively or negatively, is necessary. The professional may select from a variety of processes to promote desired change. These processes include communication, counseling, behavior modification, consultation, education, group process, supervision, administration, planning, and evaluation. Before applying change strategies, the professional should establish that the individual is an informed, willing partner.

Some people are more resistant than others to making changes in lifestyles, and such resistance to modifying their old patterns of behavior should be considered normal.[15] Change upsets the established ways of doing things, creates uncertainty and anxiety, and forces the need for adjustments. Because attitudes are thought to be the predisposing agents of practice, they should be explored. Every problem has two aspects—what the person thinks about it, and how he feels about it. Both must be considered and dealt with for problem solving and change to occur.

Although the helper may see the need for change, he should bear in mind that the client is the one who decides which changes to make and who ensures that they continue. Thus, the client's priorities take precedence over those of the professional. Evaluating the meaning of change to the individual and then motivating him to change are necessary. Those being counseled should be given an opportunity to discuss changes and to ask questions, because the more they internalize the new ideas and solutions, the greater is the likelihood of their being committed to them.

When an individual deals with the necessity of change in his food patterns and behaviors, knowledge and education are not in themselves sufficient to motivate him to change. Many people already know what they should eat, but do not act on their knowledge. The health professional cannot assume that recommendations will be followed just because the patient or client knows them. Why should any person change a lifetime of unrestricted eating that may be pleasurable? Cooperation of the patient or client is voluntary. Wanting to do what he should is a key point for the individual to consider in adopting changes in dietary practices. Motivation for change should be examined since people can be expected to resist change.[16]

Group sessions are often utilized for nutrition education and for employee communication and training. The effect of support groups on change can be either positive or negative. Face-to-face communication with someone who has successfully altered his behavior can be effective in promoting the adoption of changes by others.[17] While increasing knowledge and growing awareness may be developed in such groups, the actual change occurs through an individual's decision making.[15]

Several other factors influence success in planned change. The more communicable something is (i.e., the easier it is to describe), the more clearly it is understood. Simplicity is an advantage, as increasing complexity is associated with less readily adopted changes. The change must be compatible with the person's existing values and beliefs. If divisible into parts, a change may be tried out on a small scale so that any barriers can be worked out. The change should have a relative advantage, or be perceived as preferable in efficiency, health, pleasure, economics, prestige, and the like. Pleasure or the absence of it may change the rate of acceptance of new practices. One problem is that many of the less nutritious foods have the highest prestige value. The influence of each factor on change is a relative one. Pleasure may be a major factor in some cases, and cost or ease of food preparation an important factor in another.[18]

NUTRITIONAL COUNSELING

One aspect of nutritional care is the application of the science of nutrition to the health care of people through nutritional counseling and education. The dietitian spends a significant amount of time interacting with patients and clients. Counseling and education are essential to the maintenance of normal nutrition and health, as well as to the management of chronic diseases. Dietary practices are linked to a number of health problems, such as obesity, dental caries, cardiovascular disease, diabetes mellitus, and some types of cancer. The degree of skill in interpersonal interaction affects the quality of nutritional care provided, the degree of success or failure of the patient or client in adapting to his dietary and medical problem, and his future state of health. The following model depicts the relationship of nutritional counseling to health:[19,20]

Nutritional counseling and education	→	Changes in food intake (compliance)	→	Altered risk factors	→	Desirable health outcomes	→	Economic benefits

Nutritional counseling and education should lead to changes in food intake that alter the risk factors for disease and produce better health. Although conclusive evidence is not available to prove the first link between nutritional counseling and changes in food intake, counseling is the most reliable means of bringing about patient compliance or adherence to recommendations.[21] Economic benefits to be derived are the cost savings that result from a reduction in the incidence or severity of a disease.

The focus of the dietitian's role has shifted from the "diet instruction" of the past to the process of nutrition counseling, in which specific efforts are made to assist patients or clients in changing their eating behaviors. Formerly, the hospital dietitian, upon receipt of the physician's order for a diet instruction, taught the patient his modified diet using a printed sheet of instructions. Too often, the request was received at the last minute prior to hospital discharge, and the instruction was a one-shot, hit-or-miss situation.[22] Fifteen or 20 minutes is not sufficient time to effect significant change in an individual's eating patterns, and nutritional care is too important to health to be handled in this fashion. The ideal situation for nutrition counseling and education consists of a process over a period of time in which the client develops a growing awareness of his food intake and dietary practices, and of how these factors influence his health. The process of assisting people in establishing and maintaining good nutritional habits is a complex task, as it requires people to make permanent changes in their eating habits. Nutritional counseling and education should not be a one-time service. Follow-up counseling is an important part of care.

The amount of time required to perform nutritional services has been reported to range from 45 minutes to 12 hours or more. A consulting nutritionist employed in a corporate health office reported, for example, that initial visits lasted 45 to 60 minutes, with follow-up appointments lasting 15 to 30 minutes. As a benefit of employment, nutrition counseling was provided on company time.[23] Hatten spent 45 minutes providing initial nutrition counseling in home care services, with follow-up home visits for those who appeared to be confused or failed to understand recommendations.[24] At the Diabetes Education Center in Minneapolis, a minimum of 6 to 12 hours was the estimated time required to evaluate and educate an individual regarding diet, tailoring the diet to the client.[25] This time excludes follow-up after discharge. If the clinical dietitian has insufficient time for counseling, patients can be referred to consultant dietitians in private practice, and to community resources, for outpatient follow-up.

DIETARY ADHERENCE

Dietitians are expected to promote good dietary compliance. Compliance may be defined as the extent to which the individual's food and dietary behaviors coincide with the dietary recommendations and prescriptions. In measuring compliance, some health professionals also consider whether or not appointments are kept. Human noncompliance dates back to the Biblical story of the Garden of Eden, where Eve ate the forbidden apple from the tree of knowledge, thus associating temptation and noncompliance with guilt and sin.[26]

The term "compliance" has authoritarian overtones of a counselor deciding what is best for the individual, who is passive and compliant. The word "adherence" may suggest greater participation by the client in problem solving and decision making regarding dietary changes, which are voluntary behaviors. These terms, however, seem to be used interchangeably. The individual must adopt dietary changes and sustain them over a period of time, often a lifetime if the condition is a chronic one, such as diabetes mellitus, or cardiovascular or renal disease. The person is expected to make permanent changes to remain in optimum health. Diet may be only one of several changes the individual is expected to effect; additional changes related to his smoking, drinking, or exercise habits, together with the need to take medications, may seem overwhelming to him.

Compliance is a problem area, and some responsibility for noncompliance rests with the providers of care.[27] Although noncompliance may be viewed as failure on the patient's part to cooperate with recommendations, the counselor is not excused for other variables that are under his control, such as the quality of the client-counselor relationship and the use of appropriate influencing strategies.

Noncompliance with medical advice has been well documented. Adherence to long-term medical regimens averages about 50%, and adherence to dietary regimens is approximately 30%, with a range of 13 to 75%.[21,26] These figures suggest that some individuals abandon prescribed diets totally. In one study of dietary compliance, all patients disclosed some instances of noncompliance when questioned carefully.[28] In another report, only 2% of dietitians thought that most of their patients adhered to a prescribed diet following hospital discharge.[29] Part of the problem was that dietitians did not aggressively pursue dietary counseling while patients were in the hospital, or did not take much initiative in planning for follow-up.

It is probably unrealistic to expect 100% adherence to dietary changes every day of the week. How many people have never been tempted to stray from eating nutritionally balanced meals every day of every month, including holidays and social occasions? The fact is that most have, and thus short-term goals, such as following the diet two out of three meals daily or four days a week, may promote better adherence early in the counseling process; later, the regimen can be extended. The dietitian knows exactly what should be done and is steeped in the important reasons for dietary changes. Because he wants the patient or client to be just as knowledgeable, he runs the danger of setting unrealistic goals for change or of giving too much information at one time, accomplishing less than he would by parceling out his recommendations over time.

Factors Influencing Adherence. The many factors influencing adherence to a prescribed dietary regimen are often reported and analyzed in terms of four sets of characteristics, those belonging (1) to the patient or client, (2) to the counselor, (3) to the clinic, and (4) to the regimen.[30]

Some studies investigating demographic variables of the client, such as age, sex, socioeconomic status, marital status, and the like, have not found that demographic variables predict compliance. An exception is that better comprehension of the regimen tends to be associated with higher educational levels. Recall and comprehension by the client have been found to decrease in direct proportion to the amount of information given, probably because of supersaturation of the client with recommendations, or because of excessive anxiety on the client's part, which interferes with cognitive processes. Dispensing information over a period of time in small and manageable amounts, with repetition, should enhance recall. An imaginative combining of educational techniques, such as verbal and written instructions intermixed with visual aids, should also improve results.[30]

Satisfaction with the level of care and with the attitude of the counselor have been reported to influence adherence. Problems may result if a good rapport is not developed between the counselor and the client, with the counselor taking into consideration the person's concerns and expectations. The individual's interest level may be perfunctory, or he may fail to keep appointments. Adherence may be more satisfactory if the patient sees the same counselor at each visit, and if clear-cut communication occurs so that the individual fully understands what is best for him and what is expected of him.

The characteristics of the clinic are also important. People kept waiting for long periods of time often fail to return for future appointments. A warm and caring environment, created not only by the counselor but the entire office staff, puts the client into a frame of mind that enables him to benefit from his counseling.

The characteristics of the regimen are the most important factors in adherence. Of these, complexity is the most significant. Complexity of a regimen has been negatively associated with adherence, perhaps because of the difficulty of fitting the regimen into one's daily routine.[30] Diets encompass many of the factors associated with a higher incidence of noncompliance. According to Glanz, the factors include required changes in lifestyle, which tend to be restrictive, last a long duration or a lifetime, and interfere with family habits.[21] If other barriers exist—such as high cost of the diet, lack of access to the proper foods, or extra effort, time, and skill required in preparing the diet—the likelihood of noncompliance increases.

Often, measures of compliance are based on indirect measures. Self-reports, daily records of food intake, interviews such as diet histories and 24-hour recalls, and the dietitian's subjective rating are used to collect data. All of these methods may tend to overestimate adherence. As a result, interviewing techniques that develop good rapport and are not threatening or judgmental to the client must be utilized if the practitioner is to receive honest, accurate information about adherence to dietary regimens.[21,31] No completely reliable method of assessing adherence is available.[30]

The *Health Belief Model*, which attempts to explain preventive health behavior, was developed to interpret the decisions of people not currently suffering disease, but wishing to prevent health problems.[32] It postulates that the person's beliefs about health are determinants of his readiness to take action. The three key beliefs are (1) the extent to which the person believes that he is susceptible to contracting a disease, or resusceptible in the case of an illness from which he has recovered; (2) how serious he thinks the disease would be in affecting some of life's components; and (3) what he perceives are the benefits of a regimen in terms of reducing either susceptibility to or severity of the disease, as compared with the barriers to taking action. If the individual views taking action as unpleasant, expensive, inconvenient, or upsetting, avoidance motives may serve as barriers. Best results are obtained when readiness to act is high and when physical, psychological, financial, and other barriers are low. The model has been used to study compliant behavior.

A revised formulation of the Health Belief Model was utilized in assessing mothers' compliance with physicians' recommendations on infant feeding practices. Failure to adhere to the physician's advice was reported by almost 30% of the women. The study found that having the health-related attitude "nutrition is important" and having a "concern for health" were significantly related to compliance scores.[33]

In the Multiple Risk Factor Intervention Trial (MRFIT), groups of middle-aged men received nutritional counseling to alter food behavior in an attempt to reduce the risk of coronary heart disease. Participants were to adopt the MRFIT eating pattern, and successful dietary intervention was believed to depend on the transfer of responsibility for proper food selection to participants. In promoting adherence and assessing dietary compliance, two methods utilized were a food score and food diaries.[34,35]

Nutritionists developed a food-scoring system for participant behavioral self-monitoring based on the cholesterogenic composition of foods. Participants became versed in assessing their own food scores and could evaluate their food choices, thus providing a tool for positive reinforcement of proper food behaviors. Effective change in participants' food behaviors depended on their ability to recognize proper foods with low scores and substitute them for foods with higher scores, a process providing awareness and insight. Individual counseling encouraged the achievement of a specific guideline score. The scores became an objective means of assessing dietary adherence and understanding.[34]

A second tool for measuring adherence to the MRFIT eating pattern was a three-day food record. The food-score concept was used with these records also, and aided counseling concerning appropriate food choices and necessary changes in foods selected.

Strategies Promoting Adherence. A number of intervention strategies, including counseling, behavior modification, and education, promote improved adherence with an informed, willing client, and they should provide the client with insight into himself and his situation.[27,30,36] They are presented briefly in the following paragraphs and are discussed in more detail in later chapters of this book.

1. Establish a good interpersonal, helping relationship.

2. Provide adequate education about the dietary regime and the rationale for it. A person must know what to do in order to do it correctly. Individualize the regimen for each person, and minimize and simplify the number of changes to be made. Use a variety of techniques, such as verbal and written instructions with visual aids. Counseling should be carried out over a period of time with the same counselor, with repetition of information to ensure retention, and with provision of practice when skills need to be developed.

3. Address the individual's anxieties, determine his concerns and expectations, and try to meet them. Determine what the person thinks and how he feels about the dietary regimen. Motivation has multiple facets and is affected by the person's attitudes, beliefs, values, and opinions.

4. Set a limited number (one or two) of clear, attainable short-term goals for dietary change with the individual, and gradually increase the number of goals as he builds new skills and succeeds at new behaviors. Although the professional may want immediate perfection, people change slowly. Compromise is necessary, and short-term goals can lead eventually to long-term results.

5. Positively reinforce and reward, such as by praising, whatever the individual does correctly, no matter how small the change. Teach the person to use self-rewards. Reinforcement has a potent effect on behaviors.

6. Work with families and significant others so that they can be supportive of the dietary changes. Family members, for example, can assist with controlling the environment by purchasing and preparing proper foods.

7. Have the person keep daily records of food intake, exercise, weight, blood pressure, blood sugar, and the like. Self-monitoring has a value of its own in the person's learning and assuming responsibility for his own care, as well as in diagnosing barriers and adherence problems. Make the system easy to use, and provide feedback.

8. Negotiate written contracts for change as a tool for motivation. Include specific, positive behaviors and the rewards for accomplishment.

9. Arrange for follow-up visits. Once is not enough. Identify the factors and events contributing to nonadherence, and help the individual solve problems, setting more short-term goals for change.

10. Use support groups in which some individuals model appropriate behaviors to others. Allow for discussion and problem solving, which use higher cognitive processes.

ADMINISTRATIVE/MANAGEMENT DIETETICS

The administrative dietitian and management specialist need effective communication and education skills for personal relationships with subordinates and others on the management team in the administration of increasingly complex foodservice systems. The manager deals extensively with human resources and is expected to build good human relationships. Although one may "develop" human relations skills, there is no substitute for sincerity. A fundamental factor in interpersonal relations is the trust between the superior and the subordinate.

There are a number of interrelated management functions in which communication is important. They include staffing; employee orientation and training; leadership, including motivation, morale, and productivity; and managing change in the organization. The administrative dietitian is expected to develop communication networks, and to "utilize and maintain effective horizontal and vertical lines of communication" within the organization and the surrounding community.[37] The manager needs to be skillful in verbal and nonverbal communication, in listening to others, and in recognizing and eliminating barriers to effective communication. In a survey of dietitians with administrative responsibilities who assessed their own level of competence, the greatest mean difference between career entry and the competence required for current professional practice was found in "communication."[38]

Education skills are important in the planning, implementation, and evaluation of training programs designed to help achieve the employee's personal goals as well as organizational objectives. In staffing the organization, identified positions are filled by the use of structured interviews with applicants. The new employees selected must be oriented and trained. The manager is also responsible for continuous education of current employees and for inservice education.

Increasingly, the autocratic leadership styles of the past have been replaced by more participative approaches. Employee-centered supervisors recognize the importance of allowing more subordinate participation in decision making. One advantage is that people are more likely to accept decisions that they have participated in making. In addition, supportive and participative approaches may produce better results in terms of productivity, morale, motivation, and lessened absenteeism. Management is concerned not only with what an employee can do, but with what he will do, which depends on several forces in the work environment that influence motivation.

Effective communication skills are essential in day-to-day dealings with peers and subordinates. This type of communication is utilized, for example, in discussing with employees the goals of the organization, work that needs to be done, policies, procedures, changes, problems that may be resolved through employee counseling, and performance appraisals. Face-to-face communication with employees can have an important effect on employee attitudes and behavior.

The administrative dietitian works not only with individuals, but also with groups. Communication may be facilitated through the use of meetings and conferences. Meetings may be utilized to dispense or collect information, and for problem solving and decision making. Understanding the nature of groups and group process is essential. Knowledge of the social groupings of employees is necessary for creating conditions that will elicit cooperation and thus maximize the attainment of organizational goals.

All dietitians need to be confident of their abilities in patient/client and employee interaction. In addition to their technical competence, dietitians are expected to be skilled in interpersonal relations. With patients and clients, interviewing, counseling, and education are used to influence the behavioral outcomes of dietary regimens for the betterment of the individual's health. With subordinate employees, similar skills are used, but in different environments and for different purposes. Educational and communication theories, principles, techniques, and strategies are examined in the following chapters.

SUGGESTED ACTIVITIES

1.   Divide the group into pairs for a 10-minute walk. For the first 5 minutes, have one person close his eyes and permit himself to be guided by his partner without speaking. After 5 minutes, reverse roles and have the other person become the helper. Discuss the feelings of the helper and those of the person being helped. What were the attitudes toward helping and the feelings of trust?

2. From the dietetic practice areas mentioned in the chapter, select a specialty area of practice, and interview a dietitian or nutritionist about his responsibilities, including the use of communication skills and education skills. Share this information with peers.

3. With someone trying to make changes in food practices (such as dieting), discuss the changes and the factors influencing change, including barriers. What are the factors influencing adherence?

REFERENCES

1. Lanz, S.J.: Introduction to the Profession of Dietetics. Philadelphia, Lea & Febiger, 1983.
2. A New Look at the Profession of Dietetics. Chicago, American Dietetic Assoc., 1985.
3. Muldary, T.W.: Interpersonal Relations for Health Professionals. New York, Macmillan, 1983.
4. Baldyga, W.W.: Results from the 1981 census of the American Dietetic Association. J. Am. Diet. Assoc., *83*:343, 1983.
5. Baird, S.C., and Armstrong, R.V.L.: The A.D.A. role delineation for the field of clinical dietetics. J. Am. Diet. Assoc., *78*:370, 1981.
6. Baird, S.C., and Armstrong, R.V.L.: Role Delineation for Entry Level Clinical Dietetics. Chicago, American Dietetic Assoc., 1980.
7. Baird, S.C., and Sylvester, J.: Role Delineation and Verification for Entry-Level Positions in Community Dietetics. Chicago, American Dietetic Assoc., 1983.
8. Sims, L.S.: Identification and evaluation of competencies of public health nutritionists. Am. J. Pub. Health, *69*:1099, 1979.
9. Baird, S.C., and Sylvester, J.: Role Delineation and Verification for Entry-Level Positions in Foodservice Systems Management. Chicago, American Dietetic Assoc., 1983.
10. Ericksen, K.: Communication Skills for the Human Services. Reston, VA, Reston Publ. Co., 1979.
11. Kinlaw, D.C.: Helping Skills for Human Resource Development. San Diego, University Associates, 1981.
12. Brammer, L.M.: The Helping Relationship. Englewood Cliffs, NJ, Prentice-Hall, 1973.
13. Henderson, G.: Physician-Patient Communication. Springfield, Il, Charles C Thomas, 1981.
14. Peck, E.B.: The "professional self" and its relation to change processes. J. Am. Diet. Assoc., *69*:534, 1976.
15. Carruth, B.R., Mangel, M., and Anderson, H.L.: Assessing change-proneness and nutrition-related behaviors. J. Am. Diet. Assoc., *70*:47, 1977.
16. Mahoney, M., and Caggiula, A.: Applying behavioral methods to nutritional counseling. J. Am. Diet. Assoc., *72*:372, 1978.
17. Welch, L.B.: Planned change in nursing. Nurs. Clin. North Am., *14*:307, 1979.
18. Bryant, C.A., Courtney, A., Markesbery, B.A., and DeWalt, K.M.: The Cultural Feast. St. Paul, West Publ. Co., 1985.
19. Olendski, M.C., Tolpin, H.G., and Buckley, E.L.: Evaluating nutrition intervention in atherosclerosis. J. Am. Diet. Assoc., *79*:9, 1981.
20. Mason, M., Hallahan, I.A., Monsen, E., et al.: Requisites of advocacy. J. Am. Diet. Assoc., *80*:213, 1982.
21. Glanz, K.: Trends in Patient Compliance. Chicago, American Dietetic Assoc., 1981.
22. Wylie, J.: Growth process in nutrition counseling. J. Am. Diet. Assoc., *69*:505, 1976.
23. Seidel, M.C.: The consulting nutritionist in an employee health office. J. Am. Diet. Assoc., *82*:405, 1983.
24. Hatten, A.M.: Nutrition consultant in home care services. J. Am. Diet. Assoc., *68*:250, 1976.
25. Etzwiler, D.D.: The patient is a member of the medical team. J. Am. Diet. Assoc., *61*:421, 1972.
26. Haynes, R.B.: Introduction. *In* Compliance in Health Care. Edited by R.B. Haynes et al. Baltimore, Johns Hopkins Univ. Press, 1979.
27. Glanz, K.: Strategies for nutritional counseling. J. Am. Diet. Assoc., *74*:431, 1979.

28. Glanz, K.: Dietitians' effectiveness and patient compliance with dietary regimens. J. Am. Diet. Assoc., *75*:631, 1979.
29. Schiller, M.R.: Current hospital practices in clinical dietetics. J. Am. Diet. Assoc., *84*:1194, 1984.
30. Dunbar, J.M., and Stunkard, A.J.: Adherence to diet and drug regimen. *In* Nutrition, Lipids, and Coronary Heart Disease. Edited by R. Levy, et al. New York, Raven Press, 1979.
31. Ney, D., Stubblefield, N., and Fischer, C.: A tool for assessing compliance with a diet for diabetes. J. Am. Diet. Assoc., *82*:287, 1983.
32. Rosenstock, I.M.: Historical origins of the health belief model. Health Ed. Monographs, *2*:328, 1974.
33. Morse, W., Sims, L.S., and Guthrie, H.A.: Mothers' compliance with physicians' recommendations on infant feeding. J. Am. Diet. Assoc., *75*:140, 1979.
34. Remmell, P.S., Gorder, D.D., Hall, Y., and Tillotson, J.L.: Assessing dietary adherence in the Multiple Risk Factor Intervention Trial (MRFIT). Part I. Use of a dietary monitoring tool. J. Am. Diet. Assoc., *76*:351, 1980.
35. Remmell, P.S., and Benfari, R.C.: Assessing dietary adherence in the Multiple Risk Factor Intervention Trial (MRFIT). Part II. Food record rating as an indicator of compliance. J. Am. Diet. Assoc., *76*:357, 1980.
36. Eckerling, L., and Kohrs, M.B.: Research on compliance with diabetic regimens. J. Am. Diet. Assoc., *84*:805, 1984.
37. Position paper on the administrative dietitian. J. Am. Diet. Assoc., *67*:478, 1975.
38. Snyder, J.R., Schiller, M.R., and Smith, J.L.: A comparison of career-entry administrative competencies with skills required in practice. J. Am. Diet. Assoc., *85*:934, 1985.

2

Communication

American education has traditionally emphasized two communication skills, reading and writing, and ignored two others, speaking and listening. Consequently, many people today have grown up with the false assumption that speaking and listening are natural, that because one hears, one listens, and that because one speaks, one has speaking skills. In all of the "helping professions," speaking and listening skills correlate with the professional's effectiveness with his clients and staff.

Regardless of the physician's, nurse's, or dietitian's desire to help, if he is unable to relate well on a one-to-one basis with clients and staff, he is likely to be perceived by them as ineffective. Their trust, cooperation, and confidence are positively related to their perceptions of his caring and interest, as demonstrated through his interpersonal communication.

The dietetic literature has stressed the need for dietitians to develop communication skills, pointing out that the dietitians who develop these skills are able to establish better relationships with clients.[1,2] Effective communication can be operationally defined for dietitians as the ability to use language that is appropriate to the client's and staff's level of understanding, making sure that they have enough knowledge but are not overwhelmed; the ability to develop a relationship between himself and his clients and staff; the ability to talk to them in a way that relieves anxiety; the ability to communicate to them in a way that assures their being able to recall information actively; and the ability to provide them with feedback.

This chapter discusses communication as a process, examines its components, and points out applications for dietitians. A model of the communication process is presented and discussed, followed by an explanation of the implications of the process for the verbal, nonverbal, and listening behaviors of the dietitian. The chapter concludes with a discussion of the barriers to communication.

Possessing only an intellectual appreciation of the various communication skills is of little use. Some sciences, such as mathematics, physics, chemistry, and biology, can be mastered by learning principles; the applied social sciences cannot. Being able to pass a test by explaining how one ought to interact with clients and staff, how to defuse their hostility, and how to create a supportive communication climate with them is not the same as actually being able to do it. Putting the principles into practice requires a conscious effort, repeated attempts, and months of practice. With practice, in a relatively short time, one can notice a difference in the way others respond to him. Honing the skills, however, needs to be an ongoing process, beginning with an understanding of the many elements included in the interpersonal communication transaction.

The term "communication" is something of an enigma. Although everyone communicates, it is so expansive that it is difficult to define. In a broad sense, communication includes all methods that can convey thought or feeling between persons. The *Journal of Communication* has published no less than fifteen working definitions of human communication.[3] From among the definitions, two common elements emerge: (1) Communication is the process of sending and receiving messages. (2) For a transmission of ideas to be successful, a mutual understanding between the communicator and the listener must occur.

INTERPERSONAL COMMUNICATION MODEL

Complicated processes are easier to grasp when they can be visualized in a model. A model, however, is not the same as the actual phenomenon; rather, it is a graphic depiction to aid understanding. The elements included in the human communication model are the following: sender, receiver, the message itself—verbal and nonverbal, feedback, and interference. They are depicted graphically in Figure 2-1.

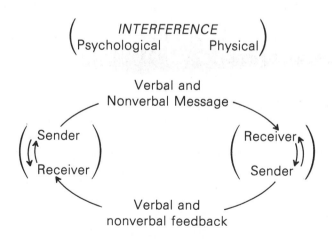

Fig. 2-1. A dietitian's communication model. (Adapted from Tindall, W. N., Beardsley, R. S., and Curtiss, F. R.: Communication in Pharmacy Practice. Philadelphia, Lea & Febiger, 1984.)

Components of the Communication Model. *Sender.* The sender of the message is the first person to speak, the one who initiates the communication.

Receiver. The receiver of the message, the listener, usually interprets and transmits simultaneously. He may be listening to what is being said and thinking about what he is going to say when the sender stops talking. Even when he is silent, it is impossible for the receiver in a two-way communication transaction not to communicate. He may be reacting physiologically with a flushed face or trembling hands, or in some other way, depending on his inferences from the message. The sender makes inferences based on the receiver's appearance and demeanor and adjusts subsequent communication accordingly.

Message. The receiver interprets two messages simultaneously: the actual verbal message and the nonverbal message inferred from the sender and the environment. Nonverbal inferences arise from the perceived emotional tone of the sender's voice, facial expression, dress, choice of words, diction, and pronunciation, as well as from the communication environment.

Feedback. The term "feedback" refers to the process of responding to messages after interpreting them for oneself. It is the key ingredient that distinguishes two-way from one-way communication. In two-way, face-to-face communication, while the sender is talking, he is looking at the other. The other's reactions to the sender's message, whether agreement, surprise, boredom, hostility, and the like, are examples of feedback.

A writer cannot clarify for readers because he doesn't see them. Even when the writer carefully selects words for the benefit of the intended reader, written communication is generally less efficient than one-to-one verbal communication because of its inability to re-explain and adjust language in response to the feedback from receivers.

Interpersonal communication, after the first few seconds, becomes a simultaneous two-way sending and receiving process. While the sender is talking, he is receiving the nonverbal reactions of the receiver. Based on these reactions, he may change his tone, speak louder, use simpler language, or in some other way adjust his communication so that his message is better understood by the receiver.

Interference. This term is used to denote the multiple factors of the communicators (sender and receiver) and of their environment that affect the interpretation of messages. These factors include the unique attributes inherent in each of them; the room size, shape, and color; temperature; furniture arrangement; and the physiological state of each communicator at the moment. The sophisticated communicator needs to understand these contingencies and to compensate for them, when possible, so that the intended message is the one received.

A crying baby, the sound of thunder, and low-flying planes, for example, not only can hinder the receiver in hearing the sender's message, but also can generate messages and interpretations in the receiver that were never intended by the sender. Another source of interference is the physiological state of the communicators at the moment. No two bodies are exactly alike. Because no one has shared in the exact life experience of another, no two people understand language in precisely the same way.

Distortions can stem from psychological interference as well, including bias, prejudice, and being closed-minded. Psychological interference in health care is often due to fear of illness and its consequences.[4] The job of the sender is to generate in the receiver those meanings for language that are closest to his own. Because meanings are not universal, they can be affected by external as well as internal influences. The communication environment, the distance between speakers, the lighting, the temperature, and colors are a few of the variables that can affect the meanings ascribed to a message. These variables can be sources of interference and major factors in accounting for the difficulty in generating in another the same meanings one has in himself. In the second half of this chapter, under the heading "Barriers to Effective Communication," additional physical and psychological forms of interference are discussed.

VERBAL AND NONVERBAL COMMUNICATION

Verbal communication includes the actual words selected by the sender and the way in which these symbols are arranged into thought units. Nonverbal communication includes the communication environment, the manner and style in which the communication is delivered, and the internal qualities inherent in the sender and receiver that influence their interpretation of external stimuli. Although verbal and nonverbal communication occur simultaneously during interaction, each is discussed separately in the context of their influence on the communication process.

To keep the communication channel open between the client or employee and the dietitian, the dietitian needs to know how to create a supportive communication climate. A supportive climate is one where as one person speaks, the other listens, attending to the message rather than to his own internal thoughts and feelings.

Although maintaining a supportive climate is always a concern, it becomes especially crucial when the professional is attempting to discuss a topic the client or employee views differently, or attempting to resolve conflict and defuse anger. The behavioral sciences offer suggestions on what one can do verbally and nonverbally to create a supportive climate under conditions of hostility or stress.[5]

Verbal Communication. The verbal guidelines for creating a supportive communication climate are to discuss problems descriptively rather than evaluatively; to describe situations with a problem orientation rather than in a manipulative way; to offer alternatives provisionally rather than dogmatically; to treat clients as equals rather than as persons of lower rank than oneself; and to be empathic rather than neutral or self-centered.

Ordinarily, when approaching topics that tend to provoke defensiveness in clients, professionals should think through the discussion prior to engaging the client, so that the problem area is exposed descriptively rather than evaluatively. Whenever one hears another judging his attitude, work, or behavior, he shows an increased tendency to become defensive. Such comments as "You don't seem to be trying," "You don't care about cooperating," or "You are selfish" are based on inferences rather than facts. So when the other says, "I do care," "I am too trying," or "I am not selfish," the framework for an argument is set, with no way of proving objectively who is right or wrong. Instead of making judgments regarding another's attitudes, the safest and least offensive way of dealing with a touchy issue is to describe the facts as objectively as possible. For example, the professional tells a client that his continuing to eat four pork chops and a half pound of chocolates a day is frustrating to him as the client's diet counselor. The professional is confronting the problem honestly and objectively without being evaluative. The client can then address the topic of his overeating rather than argue the dietitian's negative evaluation of his poor attitude, lack of concern, or noncooperativeness.

Accusing an employee who has arrived late several mornings of being "irresponsible" and "uncaring" is likely to provoke a hostile refutation or cold silence. The employee may believe that his being late doesn't warrant a reprimand. He may, in fact, have a reasonable explanation. Describing to him how his being late is frustrating, causing problems because others depend upon him, and that work has begun to back up, is honest, descriptive, and allows for nondefensive dialogue.

Orienting a person to a problem rather than manipulating him promotes a supportive communication climate. Frequently, when one wants another to appreciate his point of view, he leads him through a series of questions until the other reaches his insight. This is a form of manipulation and provokes defensiveness as soon as the respondent realizes he is being channeled to share the other's vision. It goes something like this:

"Three weeks ago I believe you told me you gained weight on the diet because your metabolism is slow, correct? Two weeks ago you told me that you gained weight because the diet itself was faulty, correct? We checked your metabolism, and it is normal, and I have assured you that someone of your size could not gain weight on 1200 calories a day. Today you tell me that you ate salty popcorn last night and that your weight gain for the third consecutive week is all water, correct? If you were dealing with a client like yourself, would you begin to get the feeling that this person is making a fool out of you?"

A discussion with this client would probably be more productive if the dietitian took a direct problem-oriented approach:

"In three weeks on a 1200-calorie diet you have gained 1 pound per week. After checking the results of your lab tests, I am certain that the diet should have caused a weight loss of 4 to 5 pounds. There seems to be problem here. Let's discuss what the other possibilities might be."

Although opening remarks should be planned descriptively rather than evaluatively, the dietitian, after making them, should allow for spontaneous problem solving without preplanned solutions. Creative, superior, and long-lasting solutions are more likely to occur when each person allows himself to hear the other out fully and be heard in return. If one is intent on "selling" a solution to the other, there is a natural disposition to block out conflicting opinions. The problem-solving process is discussed in detail in Chapters 4 and 6.

In the example of the previous paragraphs, the dietitian's subsequent remarks depend on how the client or employee responds to the directive to explain the underlying problem. The dietitian might need to wait several minutes for an answer. Providing excuses or putting words into the other's mouth is a mistake. The dietitian needs to learn the discipline of sitting through the tension of silence supportively until the client or employee responds. Frequently, the first explanations are those that people believe will not upset or shock the professional. The "real" reasons, however, may not be revealed until the client or staff member feels secure enough to risk shocking the professional without fear of being humiliated or embarrassed. After the first explanations are offered, the dietitian would do best simply to repeat in his own words what he has understood. If the client or employee is comfortable enough, he will then be able to express the reactions, questions, or answers that are less logical, more emotional, or more risky.

When offering advice to clients or helping them to solve problems, the professional should give advice provisionally rather than dogmatically. "Provisionally" implies the possibility of the dietitian's changing his opinion, *provided* additional facts emerge. It keeps the door open for the client to add information. When advice is offered in a dogmatic way, it becomes threatening for the client or employee to challenge it or add his own information. A dogmatic prescription might be, "This is what you must do. I know this is the way to solve your problem." A provisional prescription might be, "Here is one thing you might consider," or "There may be other ways of handling this problem; perhaps you have some ideas too, but this is one thing you might consider."

In discussing problems, clients and dietitians should regard each other as equals. Whenever the possibility of defensiveness exists, even between peers of equal rank, any verbal or nonverbal behavior that the other interprets as an attempt to emphasize superiority generates a defensive response. In the relationship between the dietitian and client or the dietitian and employee, the dietitian's tendency to emphasize status or rank may arise unconsciously from a desire to convince the other to accept his recommendations. Comments such as the following may cause the other to feel inferior, hurt, or angry: "As a lay person, you might not be able to grasp the theory, but it works," or "Just do what I ask; I've been doing this for ten years." Certainly, there is nothing wrong with the dietitian's letting clients know that he is trained and competent. In fact, clients often need and appreciate the reassurance. The manner in which it is done is crucial, however. A more effective and subtle way to solve problems with a client is to say, "Although I have studied this problem and dealt successfully with other clients who have similar symptoms, I am interested in incorporating your own insights and plans into our solution. You must be satisfied and will have to live with the diet, so please express your views too."

An employee making a recommendation to a dietitian that the dietitian had tried unsuccessfully himself many years ago, might be told, "If I was in your shoes, I would think the same thing. Someday when you are more experienced, you'll know why it won't work." The subtle underscoring of the inferior relative status of the subordinate could be enough to cause a defensive battle. The dietitian would have done far better with a comment such as "I can understand why you say that. I had the same idea myself. I appreciate the suggestion, but I have tried it myself unsuccessfully. Thank you." Here the employee is left feeling reinforced and appreciated rather than humiliated. Showing respect for the client's and employee's intelligence and life experience and recognizing the human dignity in the other facilitate receiving his cooperation.

In conflict resolution, problem solving, and the discussion of any issues that may be threatening to the client or employee, collaboration is far more effective than trying to persuade the individual to act according to the dictates of the professional. Collaboration has other virtues as well. People feel more obligation to uphold those solutions that they themselves have participated in designing. If the person is trying the dietitian's solution, he may feel little satisfaction in proving the dietitian was right; however, if the solution is one that they both participated in designing, there is genuine satisfaction in proving its validity. An additional reason dietitians ought to involve others in problem solving is that often a valid solution that is superior to any the individual or dietitian would have discovered alone can be arrived at through collaboration. Two people sharing insights, knowledge, experience, and feelings can generate creative thought processes in each other, which in turn generate other ideas that would not otherwise have emerged.

Another verbal skill essential to maintaining a supportive climate is the ability to empathize. Traditionally, empathy has been defined as the ability to put onself in the other's shoes. For a helping professional, however, that is not enough. To be effective in working with clients and employees, the dietitian must be able to demonstrate in some way his desire to understand what it is they are feeling. This "demonstration" might be an empathic response to their comments. In an empathic response, the listener tells the other that he is attempting to understand not only the speaker's content, but also his underlying feelings. For example, a client might say, "For my entire life I have eaten spicy foods; they are a part of my culture. I don't know what my life will be like without them." The professional might then respond, "You feel worried that the quality of your life will change because of the severe dietary restrictions."

If the dietitian is accurate in his empathic remarks, the client will acknowledge it and probably go on talking, assured that he is with a helper who listens. If the dietitian is wrong, however, the client will clarify the judgment and continue to talk, assured that he is with a helper who cares. Thus, the dietitian need not be accurate in his inferences of the other's feelings as long as he is willing to try to understand them. In addition, empathic responses allow the professional to respond without giving advice, focusing instead on the individual's need to talk and to express his feelings and concerns. Before the client or employee can listen to the dietitian, he must express all of his concerns; otherwise, while the dietitian is talking, the client or employee is thinking about what he will say when the dietitian stops.

An employee who has asked to be released from work on a busy weekend to attend a rock concert out of town might receive the following neutral response: "No offense, but a rule is a rule. If I make an exception for you, others will expect it." Alternatively, the employee would still feel sad about working but would feel less antagonistic toward the supervisor if he were to receive the following empathic response: "I realize how badly you feel about not being able to attend the concert, particularly because your girlfriend gave you the tickets as a birthday gift. I feel terrible myself having to refuse your request. I am truly sorry, but I can't afford to let you off." The supervisor, by letting the subordinate know that he has encountered him enough to pick up his underlying feelings and that he is sympathetic, uses the most effective means of defusing the subordinate's anger or antagonism. For further discussion of empathy, see Chapters 3 and 4.

Most people have not incorporated the skill of paraphrasing into their communication repertoire. Even after a person realizes how vital this step is, and begins to practice it, he may feel uncomfortable. Often the person just beginning to use paraphrasing in his inter-actions feels self-conscious and fears others may be insulted or think he is "showing off" professional communication skills. This fear itself, unfortunately, causes some people to alienate others, while trying to communicate with them. A hint for the dietitian feeling awkward about asking clients and staff to paraphrase would be to ask for the paraphrase by acknowledging his own need to verify that what he has heard is what the other intended. He might say, for example:

"I know that I don't always grasp everything immediately, and that frequently, I need to repeat what I think I have understood. My instructions today may be a bit complicated for someone who has never had to count food exchanges before. Just to be sure the instructions are understood as intended, would you mind explaining in your own words how you plan to manage this diet?"

Of course, it takes less time to ask, "Have you got it?" Asking this question is less effective, however. Because of the perceived status distinction between the helper and the person being helped, the latter may be ashamed to admit that he has not understood. Perhaps in the back of his mind, he is thinking that he can read about it later or ask the patient in the next bed for an explanation after the dietitian leaves the room. When persons of perceived higher status ask others if they "understand," almost always the answer is, "Yes." Another possibility is that the client or staff member honestly believes that he has understood, and for that reason has answered, "Yes." His understanding, however, may include some alteration of the original message, in the form of substitution, distortion, addition, or sub-traction. The skill of paraphrasing needs to become "second nature" and automatic for the professional dietitian as he verifies important instructions and significant client/staff disclosures.

Because of the anxiety attached to being in the presence of an-other of perceived higher status, the client or staff member may be less articulate than usual when describing symptoms or explaining a problem. The dietitian should paraphrase to verify that he is un-derstanding the message according to its intended meaning. The professional should avoid sounding too clinical with such comments as "What I hear you saying is . . ." or "Run that past me again"; rather, he should keep the language clear, simple, and natural. A comment such as "I want to make sure I am understanding this; let me repeat what you are saying in my own words" is more natural.

Two points need to be emphasized regarding paraphrasing. (1) Not everything the other says needs paraphrasing. It would become a distraction if, after every other sentence, the dietitian interrupted with a request to paraphrase. Paraphrasing is essential only when the discussion is centered on critical information that must be understood. (2) Paraphrasing often leads to additional disclosure and therefore tends to cause longer interaction sessions. People are so accustomed to being with others who do not really listen that when they are with someone who proves he has been paying attention by repeating the content of what has been said, they usually want to talk more. For the dietitian, this additional information can be valuable. Another benefit is that after the client or staff member has expressed all his questions and concerns and has cleared his mental agenda, he is psychologically ready to sit back and listen, or to solve problems with the dietitian. By talking too much or too soon, the dietitian may not be able to convey all of his message to the other, who may be using the difference in time between how fast the dietitian speaks and how fast his own mind processes information* to rehearse what he is going to say next.

Nonverbal Communication. Of the two messages received simultaneously by receivers, verbal and nonverbal, ordinarily it is the nonverbal that is more influential. As receivers of messages, people learn to trust their interpretations of nonverbal behavior more than the verbal word choices consciously selected by the sender. Intuitively, they know that control of nonverbal behavior is generally unconscious, while control of verbal messages is usually deliberate.

The chief nonverbal vehicles inherent in communicators are facial expression, tone of voice, eye contact, gesture, and touch. Receivers of communication perceive nonverbal behavior in clusters. Ordinarily, one does not notice posture, eye contact, or facial expression isolated from the other nonverbal channels. For that reason, professionals need to monitor all of their nonverbal communication vehicles so that together the clusters are congruent with one another as well as with the verbal messages.

Facial expression is usually the first nonverbal trait noticed in interaction. A relaxed face with pleasant expression is congruent with a supportive climate. A supportive tone of voice is one that is calm, controlled, energetic, and enthusiastic. Supportive eye contact includes gazing at the other in a way that allows the communicator to encounter the other visually—to the extent of being able to notice the other's facial and bodily messages. Besides being an excellent vehicle for feedback, eye contact also assures the other of the dietitian's interest and desire to communicate. Attending to the other visually allows inferences of interest, concern, and respect. The dietitian's posture is best when leaning somewhat toward the person as opposed to away from him. Large expansive gestures may be interpreted as a show of power and, in general, should be avoided.

---

* The human mind operates five to eight times faster than human speech.[6]

Like eye contact, touch can work positively in two ways. (1) Through a gentle touch, a pat, or a squeeze of the hand, one can communicate instantly a desire to solve a problem without offending the other. Touch can communicate affection, concern, and interest faster than these messages can be generated verbally. (2) Like eye contact, touch is a vehicle for feedback. While an individual may look calm, controlled, and totally at ease, a touch can reveal nervousness and insecurity. These clues when monitored by the dietitian, often provide insight. He reacts to them by spending more time putting the person at ease, he has the individual paraphrase to make sure the information is being understood, and he makes an effort to alter his communication style to be more overt in his support. People usually respond positively to touch, whether or not they are consciously aware of it.

Besides the dietitian's concern with the environment and his own verbal and nonverbal behavior in his attempt to create a trusting climate between himself and others, he must also be sensitive to the nonverbal cues in people. Even though the dietitian is being open, natural, caring, and attending to his own behavior and the environment, the internal anxiety, confusion, nervousness, or fear in people may be causing them to misunderstand or to react inappropriately. Two requirements for effective interpersonal communication, therefore, are that the professional observe the nonverbal cues in others and then respond to them in an affirming way.

If the client or employee is nodding his head to suggest understanding but looks puzzled, the dietitian needs to verify understanding by having the individual paraphrase important instructions or dietary recommendations. If the patient is flushed, has trembling hands, or tears rolling down his cheeks, the dietitian may need to deal directly with relieving anxiety before communicating instructions or explanations. Until the patient is relaxed enough to concentrate, optimal two-way communication between him and the dietitian is unlikely.

After talking with one another for only a few minutes, both the dietitian and the patient can sense the "warmness" or "coldness" of the other, as well as the degree of the other's "concern." Each person tends to generalize these impressions to other qualities in the other person. If the speaker has a gentle touch, pleasant expression, and looks directly into the eyes of the listener as he talks, he might be generating inferences in the listener of his being an excellent spouse, active church member, or loving mate. Once the initial positive impression has been created, the impression tends to spread into other areas not directly related to the originally observed behavior. The process can work in the reverse as well, negatively. If the dietitian does not look at the client as he talks, touches the client in a rough way, and has an unpleasant facial expression, the inferences being created now may be arrogance, lack of concern, indifference, and "coldness." Even though these initial reactions, both positive and negative, may be inaccurate, faulty first impressions are common. The helping professional might not be given a second chance to win the client's trust and cooperation; the client's inferences regarding the dietitian's concern and positive regard need to be anticipated and begun at the initial encounter.

Seeing employees daily gives the dietitian an opportunity to reinforce or alter the perceptions the other has of him. One cannot be cold, aloof, and uncaring on a daily basis, and suddenly, because it is time to conduct an appraisal or counseling session with an employee, act differently and expect to be believed. The dietitian needs to be consistent in adding positive inferences to the impressions of his staff and clients.

Not only is it important to attempt to generate concern through one's own nonverbal behavior, manner, and disposition, it is also essential to control, whenever possible, the communication environment so that it too leads to positive inferences with a minimum of "interference." Attractive offices, rooms in pastel colors, soft lighting, intimate and private space for counseling, and comfortable furniture can all add to the client's or staff member's collective perception, promoting inferences of concern.

Related indirectly to effective communication are the actual dress and physical appearance of the dietitian. Dress and appearance are usually consciously selected, and they are nonverbal communication vehicles. The female dietitian who is overly made up or too strongly scented, or the male dietitian who is wearing an earring or open shirt revealing a hairy chest, may be well meaning and competent; by their dress, however, they risk offending a more conservative person. The professional dietitian communicates his image best when clean, wearing clean and pressed clothing and only a mildly scented cologne. Because any ostentatious show of material wealth -or status tends to provoke a defensive reaction in others, items such as expensive jewelry and other valuable possessions should be omitted.

Sometimes, when dealing with a hostile client or employee, the dietitian wants to remain calm and supportive, but his body refuses to cooperate. His face may turn red, his hands may begin to shake, and his voice may become loud and threatening. If this occurs, he should acknowledge that although he wishes to resolve the problem with the individual, he is feeling defensive and realizes that this might be upsetting the person. Because the individual sees the physical manifestations of the dietitian's defensiveness, the dietitian should acknowledge the reaction rather than attempt to feign control. Under these circumstances, the dietitian should avoid further immediate communication and should schedule another appointment after regaining composure.

Among the requirements for effective interpersonal communication is the need for the dietitian to send verbal and nonverbal messages that are congruent with one another. If a client hears a dietitian say, "I want to help you; I'm concerned about your health and any possible recurrence of your heart problem as a result of improper diet," but at the same time sees the dietitian looking down at his notes rather than at him, making no attempt to connect with him physically through handshake or gentle touch, or looking frequently at his watch, the incongruous second message of impersonality or impatience will be more intense than the stated message of concern. Although the professional has said all the "right" words, he is still judged as insincere.

Helping professionals and managers who do not genuinely like working with people are destined ultimately to fail; often, however, professionals who do like people and care for their clients and employees fail as well. To be successful in working with others, the dietitian must develop congruent verbal and nonverbal communication skills. One can develop all the appropriate verbal skills and still be unsuccessful in calming a hostile employee or client or in increasing an obstinate client's adherence to the dietary plan.

LISTENING SKILLS

Well-developed listening skills are an essential requirement for effective interpersonal communication between the dietitian and his client and staff. An individual with average intelligence can process information at speeds that are approximately five times that of human speech. The higher the intelligence is, the faster the mind tends to process information. Some individuals can think at speeds of eight to ten times the rate of human speech. Thus, while the dietitian is listening to his client or staff member talk, he has time to be thinking about other things simultaneously. Everyone has had the experience of listening to a speaker and thinking about what he might be like as a person or letting the mind wander to other topics. From the speaker's clothes, shoes, jewelry, diction, speech patterns, etc., people tend to fill in details and develop an elaborate scenario while they listen, more or less, to his presentation. The process of good listening involves learning to harness one's attention so that one is able to concentrate totally on the speaker's message, both verbal and nonverbal. Development of these skills is not difficult, but it does require a conscious effort and perseverance.

Listening is taught as an academic subject in the department of communication studies in most colleges and univesities. Research projects conducted at the University of Minnesota, however, indicate that listening ability can be enriched only when the individual desires such enrichment and is willing to follow the training with practice.[6] The following list of four of the most common poor listening habits is an excellent starting place for the reader who desires practice to improve his listening skills:[3]

1. People tend to stop listening when they have decided that the material is uninteresting and tend to pay attention only to material they "like" or see an immediate benefit in knowing.
2. Most people have a limited and undeveloped attention span.
3. Listeners tend to trust their intuition regarding the speaker's credibility, making judgments from nonverbal behavior rather than from the content of the message.
4. Listeners tend to attach too much credibility to messages heard on electronic media—radio, television, movies, tapes, etc.

Listening can be improved with practice. The most important step in such improvement is resolving to listen more efficiently. Simply being motivated to listen causes one to be more alert and active as a receiver. The following are specific suggestions for improving listening:[3]

1. Prior to engaging in the communication transaction, the listener should remind himself of his intent to listen carefully.
2. The communication situation should be approached with the attitude of objectivity, with an open mind, and with a spirit of inquiry.
3. Listeners need to watch for clues. Just as one uses bold type and italics in writing, speakers use physical arrangement, program outlines, voice inflection, rate, emphasis, voice quality, and bodily actions as aids to help the listener determine the meaning of what is being said and what the speaker believes is most important.
4. Listeners need to make use of the thinking-speaking time difference and to remind themselves to concentrate on the speaker's message. They must use the extra time to think critically about the message, to relate it to what they already know, to consider the logic of the arguments, and to notice the accompanying nonverbal behavior—all simultaneously.
5. Listeners need to look beyond the actual words to determine what the speaker means, and to determine whether the clusters of accompanying nonverbal behavior are congruent with the verbal message.

6. Listeners need to provide feedback to the speaker, either indirectly through nonverbal reactions or directly through paraphrasing, to verify that what is being understood by the listener is what the speaker intends.

7. Ultimately, the most valuable listening skill is ongoing practice. One who wants to improve his listening must put himself in difficult listening situations, must concentrate, and must practice good listening.

BARRIERS TO EFFECTIVE COMMUNICATION

Thus far this chapter has dealt with what dietitians can do verbally and nonverbally to ensure accurate communication with others. Because most people have not studied the communication process in detail, they tend to underestimate the forces and variables likely to impede the process. There are myriads of barriers that often alter perceptions, increasing the likelihood of inaccurate communication. Only after the individual is aware of these barriers can he begin to alter his communication to safeguard against them.

The major barrier to communication, which probably accounts for about 90% of the misunderstandings between people, is based on the communication principle that meanings are in people, not words. Communication scholars have been attempting to make people aware of the implications of this principle for over four decades; however, it does not yet seem to be accepted and understood by most communicators. To comprehend the principle, one needs to understand the many ways in which humans differ one from another and how these differences account for the variations in the way they understand and use language. With the possible exception of identical twins at birth, no two people have the exact same physiological make-up. While one may think that he is experiencing objective reality as he moves from one life experience to another, he is in fact interpreting objective reality subjectively through his body and mind.

To understand this point better, the reader can try to remember a time when he was not feeling like himself, a time perhaps when he was under strong medication or severe stress. If the medication or stress accelerated the processes of his nervous system, he noticed that he was more nervous, less tolerant, and perhaps more depressed than usual. If the medication slowed down these processes, he noticed that he was more lethargic, less enthusiastic, and less motivated than usual. In both cases, the objective reality would be interpreted differently than if he were in his normal state. The "normal" range varies considerably. For some, being lethargic, moody, and slow-moving is normal. For others, being energetic, hyperactive, and tireless is normal. These two "normal" individuals might attend the same party, get married, or be involved in a helping relationship.

Eventually, they will discover that each tends to interpret the same reality differently, with each assuming his interpretation is "correct."

In addition to an understanding and appreciation of the uniqueness of each person's physiological profile, there is a need to consider that over time, even the same person experiences a range of sensation, which affects inferences about reality. As people grow older, their senses change and begin to atrophy. Two people sitting at a baseball game eating hot dogs might be having different sensual experiences. One is enjoying and savoring every mouthful, while the other is lamenting, "They just don't make them like they used to." The senses of sight, hearing, touch, smell, and taste all diminish over time. These internal changes add to the problem of inferring that because two people have heard the same message or shared the same experience, they therefore have the same "meanings" in their interpretation.

Two people of identical intelligence may interpret the same external stimuli differently. Some people are dispositionally oriented toward seeing details, are introverted, and are less emotional, while others with similar intelligence tend to miss details, are more extroverted, and are more emotional. Although it is usually easier to communicate with someone who is cognitively similar to oneself, intelligence alone is not a predictor of ease of communication between individuals.

Culturally, people differ from one another, which causes them to have different interpretations of the same phenomenon. One of the authors is a second-generation Italian-American. When he traveled in Italy as a young student, he understood what it meant to be an Italian-American as opposed to a native Italian. He saw the world differently from his Italian-born cousins. Although he had never examined or challenged his values, he now realized what it meant to be "acculturated." The kind of home in which a person is brought up and the values he learns as a child continue to influence the way in which he interprets the world.

Many writers have pointed out the advantages of writing in English, the language with more extant words than any other. Theoretically, the extra number of words ought to allow writers and speakers of English to express "meanings" more precisely than communicators using other languages. When the language is examined carefully, however, other limiting variables emerge. No language in the history of the world has as many words to express extremes. There are dozens of synonyms for "bad," "terrible," "evil," and "horrible," as well as of "good," "beautiful," "wonderful," "terrific," and "fantastic." English has, however, only a scant representation of words that describe intermediate feelings and thoughts, middle-of-the road positions, and other "gray" areas.

Philosophers have pointed out that thoughts are controlled to a great extent by vocabulary. One cannot think about something if one has no words for it. The inability to verbalize vague or intermediate areas of thought or feeling may distort one's perceptions of objective reality, increasing one's tendency to overreact, and hindering the likelihood of easy collaboration.

Another idiosyncrasy of the English language involves its many words with multiple meanings. The *Oxford English Dictionary*, for example, includes some 15 definitions for the word "fast." A "fast" horse, for example, is one that runs with great speed, while a "fast" color is one that does not run at all.

Generating one's own meanings in others, which involves trying to juxtapose meanings so that one can arouse his exact meanings, is an extremely difficult process. Because we are each unique physiologically, psychologically, socially, and culturally, and because we speak a language that is susceptible to many interpretations, the process of communicating accurately to one another is complicated.

In addition to the variables previously discussed, numerous other phenomena affect the accuracy of person-to-person transmission of messages. One such factor evolves from the predictable phenomena of substitution, addition, and simplification that occur as messages are passed from person to person. As messages are sent from sender to receiver, each receiver tends to alter the message unconsciously when he becomes a sender and passes it on to another.

While distortion of messages are predictable, additional complications arise from status distinctions between the interactants. When someone who has the power to reward or punish another attempts to give instructions, teach a procedure, or merely relate a series of facts, his perceived higher status often makes understanding the message more difficult for the receiver who perceives himself to be of lower status.

Sensations similar to the tension, stress, and side effects of the adrenal secretions of prehistoric humans fighting for survival still exist in people today. When an employee is called before his boss, who wishes to explain the importance of the employee's task or a complicated procedure, the employee might become nervous, experience trembling hands, begin to perspire, feel his face become flushed, or develop the feeling of "butterflies" in his stomach. These "fight-or-flight" symptoms often make it even more difficult to think clearly. At the very time when one needs to be most alert, he may be subject to a physiological handicap.

The most salient implication for the dietitian engaged in helping clients or training staff is the need to compensate for this phenomenon by assisting his clients and employees in developing the appreciation and ability of paraphrasing. In the presence of health professionals, clients and staff members often experience tension and anxiety, which make it difficult for them to grasp messages. The dietitian needs to learn communication skills to compensate for this tendency. In addition to being natural, deemphasizing status distinctions, using clear, concise language, and showing concern, the dietitian must consistently paraphrase the other, as well as have himself paraphrased, to verify that what was explained or taught was understood.

A final barrier to communication is the human tendency to perceive information selectively, and to be intolerant of others who interpret the information differently. General Motors, for example, did a study several years ago to determine who reads Pontiac advertisements. The corporation learned that the major consumers of information about Pontiac automobiles are Pontiac owners. Each person tends to tune in to information that supports his already existing attitude and tends either to distort or not to hear information that refutes his existing attitudes.

Count the "F's" in the following statement:

FASCINATING FAIRYTALES ARE THE
RESULT OF YEARS OF SCIENTIFIC
STUDY COMBINED WITH THE
EXPERIENCE OF CREATIVE MINDS.

Most people looking at the message above for the first time, and told to count the number of "F's" see three. Even after being told that there are actually six, some people continue to see only three. How many do you see? Although many people believe themselves to be open-minded, unprejudiced, and able to see all sides of an issue, this simple test provides some evidence that there is the tendency in each of us to lock onto an expected view of reality and miss the objective truth.

This tendency to perceive reality selectively is unconscious. In general, people are unaware of which stimuli their minds are selecting to attend to and which stimuli are being ignored. For this reason, stereotypes, biases, and prejudices are likely to emerge and distort interpretations of messages. Such distortions carry implications for professional dietitians. In dealing with clients or staff members, they must consciously attempt to verify perceptions as a safeguard against selective distortion. One of the best ways to accomplish this is to listen actively, paraphrasing and making empathic responses. If the empathic response or paraphrasing is inaccurate and represents selective perception, the other person has the opportunity to clarify.

Nothing is as frightening to humans as the fear of uncertainty and ambiguity. When a person has the opportunity to try out new communication behavior, forces within him tend to pull him toward his past behavior. Even if his old methods have been unsuccessful, he is comforted by their producing predictable results.

This chapter has presented numerous suggestions for improving the dietitian's communication competence with clients and staff. One can read and reread this chapter, pass a quiz on the material with a grade of A⁺, and still be ineffective in practicing communication skills. To develop communication skills, the reader must begin immediately to put into practice what he has read. He should not be discouraged if he cannot employ all skills immediately. Months of conscious attention to these skills are needed before they become a part of one's natural approach to clients and staff.

The dietitian who is serious about increasing his communication competence needs to swallow hard and stretch, forcing himself to attempt the new behavior. The time to begin is *now*. One need not have access to clients or staff. One can exercise these skills just as effectively in his personal as in his professional life. Despite all the problems, improved communication is possible, and the professional who is aware of the problems and the safeguards to them is more effective.

SUGGESTED ACTIVITIES

1. After filling out the questions below, join with classmates in groups of three to share and discuss your responses with one another.

A. What types of nonverbal signals from your instructor or supervisor indicate to you that he is getting angry?

    a.

    b.

    c.

B. What nonverbal cues indicate that you are getting angry?

    a.

    b.

    c.

C. List some of the nonverbal signals that you send when you are talking and someone interrupts you.

    a.

    b.

    c.

D. List some of the nonverbal signals you send when you want to signal confidence or approval of the other person.

    a.

b.

c.

E. List changes you might make in the room where you are reading to alter its climate positively.

a.

b.

c.

2. Write a two-paragraph description of a current interpersonal conflict you are experiencing. Be sure to indicate (1) the behavior on the part of the other that has caused you a problem and (2) what "feelings" you are experiencing as a result of that behavior. Do not sign your name unless you want to be acknowledged. After the instructor has collected the descriptions, he may read them and either invite students to participate in role-playing of the situations, using the guidelines for supportive verbal and nonverbal behavior, or engage the class in a case study discussion of how the communication skills might be employed to resolve the conflict.

3. The following is an exercise that the reader might try with friends. The first person expresses the message to the second, who in turn expresses it to the third, and so on until six people have heard it. Ordinarily, the message is audiotaped and played back. This allows the participants to see the many ways in which messages are altered as they pass from person to person.

Message:

There has been an accident, and I must report it to the police. It is necessary, however, for me to get to the hospital as soon as possible.

The cement truck, heading east, was turning left at the intersection when the sports car, heading west, attempted to turn right. When they saw that they were turning into the same lane, both honked their horns, but each continued to turn without slowing down. Actually, the truck appeared to be speeding up just before the crash.

REFERENCES

1. Owen, A.: Challenges for dietitians in a high tech/high touch society. J. Am. Diet. Assoc., *84*:285, 1984.
2. Eckerling, L., and Kohrs, M.: Research on compliance with diabetic regimens—Applications to practice. J. Am. Diet. Assoc., *84*:805, 1984.
3. Samovar, L., and Mills, J.: Oral Communication, Message and Response. Dubuque, IA, William C. Brown Company, 1986.
4. Tindall, W., Beardsley, R., and Curtiss, F.: Communication in Pharmacy Practice. Philadelphia, Lea & Febiger, 1984.
5. Gibb, J.: Defensive communication. J. of Communication, *11*:141, 1961.
6. Nichols, R., and Stevens, L.: Are You Listening? New York, McGraw-Hill, 1957.

3

Interviewing

Most people have engaged in the interviewing process at one time or another. A person applying for a new position interviews the employer concerning the job opening, and in turn is interviewed by the employer. Interviewing is a skill used frequently in some occupations, such as health professions. When one seeks medical care, the physician takes a medical history using interviewing techniques. The client or hospitalized patient may be interviewed at great length and by more than one person. A considerable amount of time is spent in gaining information from an individual in order to advise, counsel, or assist him. Dietitians apply interviewing skills with patients, clients, and employees.

Interviewing may be defined as a guided communication process between two people with a predetermined purpose and an exchanging or obtaining of specific information. The interview is more than a question-and-answer session, although questions are the means of determining the subject matter of the interview. The goal of the interview is to collect valid data from the respondent while maintaining an interpersonal environment conducive to disclosure. These data include both rational and emotional reactions of the respondent.

Development of interviewing skills requires practice and repetition over time. Anyone conducting an interview for the first time may expect to feel quite uncomfortable. While some advance planning regarding the content and process of interviews is important, the warm human relationship that develops between two people differs each time, and no two interviews are exactly alike. Knowing the principles and process of interviewing, using them, and frequently evaluating their results can help students and practitioners to improve their skills. Developing listening skills is also important, as an effective interviewer must be a good listener. Skillfull listening requires concentration on the verbal and nonverbal behavior and perception of what is important in the respondent's behavior. One listens not only for facts, but also for attitudes and values.

This chapter examines the principles and process of interviews, the conditions that facilitate interviews, the three parts of an interview, the use of different types of questions, and the types of interviewer responses.

TYPES OF INTERVIEWS

For the purpose of illustrating the interviewing principles and process, two examples of interviews are referred to in this chapter— the diet history and the pre-employment interview. Although a full delineation of the content of these types of interviews is beyond the scope of this book, a brief explanation of each type follows. For more detailed information on content, other sources should be examined.[1-6]

A diet history obtained by interview is an account of a person's food habits, preferences, eating behaviors, and other factors influencing food intake. (A diet history form is presented in Appendix A.) It may be used along with other data to assess the nutritional status of the individual or may be used prior to nutritional counseling. Approaches utilized frequently are the 24-hour recall, the record of usual daily food intake, and the food frequency check.

In the 24-hour recall, the dietitian asks the client to recount in detail, qualitatively and quantitatively, all foods and beverages consumed in the previous 24-hour period. The second method, the usual daily food intake, elicits a record of what the client usually consumes during one day. In both approaches, the portion sizes, the methods of food preparation, the between-meal snacks, the times of day when food is consumed, and alcoholic beverages require consideration. Neither method is considered to have a high degree of accuracy in assessing the nutritional status of the individual, and each suffers certain deficiencies. For example, the previous 24-hour period may not have been typical of what the person normally eats, and the usual daily intake this week may differ considerably from previous weeks and may undergo seasonal variations. An additional point is that the food intake for Mondays through Fridays often differs from that of weekends. One method to increase the accuracy of the diet history is to conduct a food frequency check. A food frequency check determines the daily or weekly frequency of consuming basic foods, such as meats, milk, breads, cereals, fruits, and vegetables. With the previously mentioned methods, skillful interviewing obtains more accurate and usable information than unskilled interviewing.

In personnel management, the dietitian uses interviewing skills with prospective employees. Several applicants for the same position may be interviewed to obtain information on which to base the hiring decision. The same basic interviewing principles are utilized, but for a different purpose. Federal legislation outlaws discrimination in hiring based on race, color, religion, national origin, sex, age, and physical handicap. Those responsible for pre-employment interviews should consult other resources to determine the content of questions that may be considered discriminatory.[1-4]

PURPOSE OF THE INTERVIEW

Prior to the interview, the purpose should be clearly identified and communicated. A diet history may serve one of several purposes. The dietitian may use it as a basis for calculating the individual's daily nutrient intake, comparing it with anthropometric and laboratory data in nutritional assessment. It may be initiated by a dietitian who has identified a patient as being at high risk for nutritional deficiencies. The history may be used prior to initiating nutrition education to identify what nutritional problems the client has, and to provide a baseline for gauging change. A history can also help to determine a person's current food habits and the necessary changes when instituting counseling on a modified diet, such as a sodium-restricted diet.

In the case of a job opening, the purpose of the interview is to determine which applicant best meets the qualifications for the position, and whether the opening is suited to the person's talents. The decision of which applicant to hire is based on the interview and on other sources of information, such as the application form, references, and physical examination. A secondary purpose is to give the applicant information about the position and the organization on which to base his own decision regarding possible employment with the company. The interviewer both gives and gathers information.

The dietitian should communicate the purpose of the interview to the interviewee. With clients and patients, one can also stress that the interview is necessary to provide better advice, service, or health care to the individual, and with job applicants, that it is important to find an employee who will be satisfied with the company and the position. If the purpose is clear and understood, better cooperation from the interviewee may be anticipated.

CONDITIONS FACILITATING THE INTERVIEW

Bernstein described five conditions for effective interviewing: (1) attentiveness including attention to nonverbal behavior, (2) rapport, (3) freedom from interruption, (4) psychologic privacy, and (5) emotional objectivity.[7] In addition, the impact of physical surroundings, of the personal context of the respondent, and of note-taking should be considered.

Attentiveness. Attentive listening helps to create a climate in which the interviewee can communicate more easily. The professional needs to develop listening skills and to listen with empathy rather than to talk extensively. Listening is an active, not a passive, skill. The professional assists the interviewee in gathering and communicating his thoughts and feelings. To understand the complete message, the interviewer must listen to the verbal message while observing the nonverbal behavior, such as facial expressions and tone of voice. At the same time, the interviewee observes the nonverbal behavior of the interviewer. Frequent looking at one's watch, failure to maintain eye contact, sitting back in too relaxed a posture, frowning, yawning, and tone of voice all convey a negative message.

Rapport. Rapport should be established early in the interview. Rapport is the personal relationship established between the interviewer and the respondent and is a key to a good interview. It deals with emotional aspects, the building of a warm and supportive climate, the release of stress, and the smooth flow of conversation in a nonjudgmental atmosphere. The interviewee should be put at ease and relieved of anxiety and uncertainty of what is planned, since people react more favorably in situations that they understand and accept. Nonverbal behaviors include smiling when appropriate, having an approving facial expression, nodding approval, giving undivided attention, speaking confidently, and making people feel that one is interested in what they are saying. When the individual has been seen previously, less time may be needed to develop rapport, and a comment on something from a previous visit may be sufficient. Excessive deference, although it may be flattering to the professional, may actually inhibit development of rapport with patients. The patient, overwhelmed by the professional's expertise, may give information he thinks is being sought instead of medically useful information. Building trust in the relationship is the key to rapport.

If the person has been kept waiting for a long time, negative feelings may occur, and the person may appear angry, belligerent, or unfriendly. Recognizing that these emotions interfere with establishing a good relationship, the dietitian should apologize and attempt to reduce these feelings by saying, for example, "I'm sorry you had to wait so long. I was busy with another patient and it took longer than I expected. I can understand if you are annoyed."

Addressing people by their first names, a practice usually restricted to close friends and family, may be interpreted as lack of respect by some people, especially those who like the tradition of formal address or who are older, and this may inhibit the building of rapport. When in doubt, the dietitian should use both names, such as "John Smith" or "Mr. Smith." A first name should be used only with permission of the interviewee, after an inquiry such as "Do you prefer to be addressed as "John" or as "Mr. Smith?"[8] Using the person's preferred name does not show excessive concern with tradition, but is simply another tool for promoting rapport.

Freedom From Interruptions. Freedom from interruption furthers the impression that one is genuinely concerned about the person being interviewed. The dietitian should arrange to have phone calls held, and if a phone call should come despite such an arrangement, the dietitian should explain to the caller that a conference is in progress, and should ask the caller to return the call later. The dietitian should apologize for the interruption on hanging up, and then resume the interview.

Psychologic Privacy. Psychologic privacy is enhanced by geographic privacy, but is not absolutely necessary for psychologic privacy to exist. Since they may discuss private matters, the interviewer and interviewee should be alone. A quiet office without interruption is preferable, but at the patient's bedside in a hospital setting, others may be present in the room. Whenever possible, arrange the setting so that the interview cannot be overheard, is not interrupted, and promotes the giving of undivided attention. The interviewee should understand that what he says will not be repeated later. In a professional relationship, the confidentiality of patient, client, and applicant information must be respected. Anecdotes and stories should not be shared with others over coffee breaks, lunch, or at social gatherings.

Other variables related to the location of interviews include comfort, distance between parties, and seating arrangements. These may either help or hinder an interview, and may or may not make the other person feel more like communicating. Comfort concerns proper furniture, lighting, temperature, ventilation, and pleasant surroundings. A comfortable setting where eye contact can be maintained should be arranged. Preferably, the parties should be at the same head level, since the dietitian's standing over a patient lying in bed may trigger deferential behavior.[8] According to Stewart, the optimum distance between people involved in an interview is 3 or 4 feet, or about an arm's length.[9] The most formal seating arrangement is for one person to sit across the desk from the other, while a chair along the side of the desk is less formal and makes people feel equal in status to one another. Two parties seated without a table is informal, but when it is necessary to view materials, a round table is less formal since it avoids the head-of-the-table position. In general, the fewer the furniture barriers, the better. A clean desk top also removes distractions.

Emotional Objectivity. Emotional objectivity is another essential requirement for effective interviewing. Personal feelings and preferences should be controlled and not revealed to the interviewee. The client should feel free to express all of his feelings and attitudes and, in the process, may express some that are contrary to those of the professional. An attitude of acceptance, self-control, and concern for the interviewee should be maintained, with a desire to understand behavior, rather than to judge it.

Interviewers should be aware that a professional relationship is most easily established with persons of similar socioeconomic status, ethnic group, and possibly age, while barriers to this relationship may arise when these factors differ. The professional needs to learn about, understand, and accept the cultural differences, value systems, and lifestyles of other groups. Exploration of one's own attitudes towards those who are different may be necessary. The interviewee should feel free to discuss all matters without fear of condemnation, since any such expression blocks the progress of the interview. A raised eyebrow, a look of shock or surprise, or an incredulous follow-up question (e.g., "You had *three* pieces of pie and *two* milkshakes for lunch?") may cause the interviewee to change or to end his story. The dietitian should seek to understand the circumstances, not to pass judgment on them. If, in the interview, the respondent does not find the professional an understanding person, he is unlikely to converse freely with him.

Interviewers should develop an awareness of their own conscious and unconscious prejudices. These include not only racial or religious preferences, but also exaggerated dislikes of people and their characteristics, such as obese people, poorly dressed people, aggressive women, meek men, highly pitched voices, redheads, weak handshakes, or uneducated people. Interviewers who identify their areas of intolerance may be better able to control their expression and avoid nonverbal behaviors revealing prejudices.

Personal Context. The interviewee brings to the interview his own personal context or system of beliefs, attitudes, feelings, and values, which must be recognized.[8] Concerns about perceived threats to health can be so frightening, for example, that they preoccupy and block conversation. The dietitian would do well to recognize that the respondent's situation may have both subjective and objective aspects. That a man has had a heart attack is a medical fact, but his subjective feelings about his illness may be equally important. Fear, resentment, anger, anxiety, dependence, or regression may be underlying emotions that interfere with cooperation. The dietitian's understanding of the psychological reactions to illness and ways of dealing with them may be necessary, and a sense of caring and concern is helpful. The dietitian may need to facilitate the venting of feelings and to acknowledge them before going on to the interview.[8] A job applicant may have been laid off recently from a position that he had held for ten years, which is a fact. The subjective way he feels about his situation, however, is as important as the situation itself. Anxiety, nervousness, and depression may be evident. The dietitian should be alert for nonverbal and verbal clues about the person that provide a frame of reference for understanding.

Usually, the dietitian has some information about the person in advance, which may prove helpful in understanding the personal context of the interviewee. In the hospital setting, the medical record is a source of information on the social and economic circumstances that may influence the treatment—marital status, number in household, age, occupation, economic status, religion, level of education, physical health and activity, medications, and medical history. In pre-employment interviews, the application form should be examined in advance, since it contains information on education and previous work experience.

The professional should keep in mind that the person may be suffering from problems of which he is not consciously aware or problems that he is unable to express. The job applicant may be nervous or apprehensive about the impression he is making. The patient may be worried about his medical problem and how it will affect his future work or lifestyle. While the dietitian may be focusing on obtaining a diet history and giving diet instructions, the patient may be thinking about adjusting to his new disease or completing arrangements for hospital discharge by 2:00 P.M. By putting the person at ease, by encouraging him to talk freely, and by assisting him to organize his thoughts and feelings, the empathic, skilled listener may ease these problems.

Note-Taking. Another factor to consider is the impact of note-taking. The inexperienced interviewer may find it necessary to take notes, which may raise suspicion on the part of the interviewee and hamper the flow of communication. To avoid such concern, the dietitian should ask for the interviewee's permission to jot down a few notes, and should explain why they are necessary and how they will be used. The dietitian can ask, for example, "Is it all right if I take a few notes so that later I can review what we said?" Writing constantly throughout an interview interferes with both parties. The interviewee may become distracted, and the professional has less time for listening carefully and developing continued rapport with the person. Attention should be concentrated on what is said, not on writing. Notes should be as brief as possible, and eye contact with the interviewee should be maintained while writing. Interviewers should train themselves to remember conversations from a limited number of key words, phrases, or abbreviations. A breakfast of orange juice, cereal, toast, and coffee with cream and sugar, for example, may be abbreviated as "OJ, cer, tst, C-C-S," while a pineapple cottage cheese salad may be noted as "P/A-CC sld." Taking brief notes during an interview may be difficult for students who are accustomed to taking notes during classroom lectures, sitting passively and filling notebooks with what is said; however, this skill can be developed with time. Comprehensive notes should be dictated or written immediately at the close of the interview after the person has departed. Waiting 15 minutes or longer, seeing another client, or accepting phone calls may cause the interviewer to forget essential information.

PARTS OF THE INTERVIEW

Each interview has three parts. The initial phase or opening involves introductions and establishment of *rapport,* a process of creating trust and good will between the parties.[9] The middle phase includes asking questions to obtain information while maintaining the personal relationship, as the interviewer guides and directs the interview with responses. In the final phase, the interview is closed, and any future contacts are planned.

Opening

The opening sets the tone of the interview—friendly or unfriendly, professional or informal, relaxed or tense, leisurely or rushed. Introductions may establish several of these conditions. Interviewers should greet the client, and state first their name and job title, e.g., "Good morning. I'm Judy Jones, a registered dietitian." Eye contact, a smile, a handshake or placing a hand on the other's hand or arm, and a friendly face and tone of voice are supporting nonverbal behaviors. It is possible to be professional without being cold, distant, and formal. In the hospital setting, it may be necessary to verify who the patient is. The dietitian may ask, "Are you John Johnson?" If answered affirmatively, he may respond, "I'm glad to meet you, Mr. Johnson." If the person's physician has requested the contact, the dietitian may mention this. "Did Dr. Smith tell you that he asked me to visit you?" If the client answers, "No," the dietitian should verify the fact that the physician requested the contact. A discussion of the nature and purpose of the interview may follow, along with an explanation of how the interviewee will benefit from the interview. Stating one's name and immediately unleashing a barrage of questions should be avoided.

Discussion initially may center on known information from the medical record of patients or from the application form of job applicants. Alternatively, the weather, baseball scores, a national or international event, or any topic of joint interest may be appropriate for opening the discussion. If he perceives this conversation to be artificial or merely small talk, however, the interviewee may become tense.

When the interviewee has initiated the appointment, it is preferable to let him state in his own words his problem or his purpose for coming. The dietitian may ask him, "What brought you to the Friendly Company to seek employment?" or "How have things been goind since we last talked?" or "When we talked on the phone, you mentioned that your doctor told you that you have borderline diabetes." When the interviewee is given the chance to express himself first, the interview begins with his agenda, which is preferable.

Although it may be time-consuming for the busy dietitian, the opening exchange of either information or pleasantries is important and should not be omitted. Rapport, a degree of warmth, a supportive atmosphere, and a sense of mutual involvement are helpful to establish.[9] Willingness to disclose information about oneself is influenced by the level of trust established in the relationship, and cooperation and disclosure are crucial to the success of interviews. The interviewee quickly develops his own perceptions of the situation and makes decisions about the amount and kind of information he will share. He forms impressions of the dietitian just as the professional does of him. The purpose of the interview should be clearly stated prior to directing the conversation to the second stage.

Middle Phase

In the second stage, the interviewee is asked a series of questions. A good interviewer has preplanned and prepared an "interview guide," an outline of information desired or topics to be covered. The guide should specify not only what questions will be asked, but also how questions will be phrased in order to elicit the most information in the least amount of time. Topics should be arranged in a definite sequence. In a diet history, for example, the interviewer may desire information about beverages consumed, eating in restaurants, portion sizes, meals, methods of food preparation, and snacks. Arranged in sequence, the list includes meals, portion sizes, methods of food preparation, snacks, beverages, and eating in restaurants. In a preemployment interview, the sequence may be previous work experience, education, present activities and interests that are job-related, and personal qualifications.

While it ensures that information is gathered in a systematic manner, the interview guide does not have to be followed strictly. The interviewer should be thoroughly familiar with the questions and not have to refer to them constantly. Knowing the purpose and significance of each question is important so that questions are not asked in a perfunctory manner, and so that the interviewer does not accept superficial or inadequate answers. Asking a job applicant about offices held in organizations, for example, is an attempt to seek information about leadership ability and the acceptance of responsibility, while inquiring what he plans to be doing 5 years hence is an attempt to learn about short- and long-range goals.[10] To answer fully, the interviewee must see how the questions are relevant to his needs. With patients or clients, the dietitian can explain that the answers to questions are a basis for nutritional counseling or education. Appendix B contains supplementary information on questioning.

Using Questions. Questions play a major role in interviews. The wording of questions in interviews is important as well as one's manner and tone of voice. A friendly approach in asking the questions communicates the desire to understand and be of assistance. The kind of questions asked should require the other person to talk 60 to 70% of the time. Questions that are highly specific or that may be answered with one word or with "Yes" or "No" should be avoided initially, but may be necessary later to follow up on specific circumstances. Knowledge of the kinds of questions to use and skill in using them are important to successful interviewing. Stewart classifies questions in three ways: open or closed, primary or secondary, and neutral or leading.[9]

Open and Closed Questions. Open questions are broad and give the interviewee great freedom in responding while giving the professional an opportunity to listen and observe. Examples of open questions are:

"Can you tell me a little about yourself?"
"Can you tell me about your eating habits?"

At the beginning of the interview, open questions are less threatening, communicate more interest and trust, and reveal what the interviewee thinks is most important. Disadvantages are that they may involve a greater amount of time consumed, the collection of unnecessary information, and lengthy, disorganized answers.

Also open, but with moderate restrictions, are the following:

"What about your meals?"
"What diet have you been following?"
"What did the doctor tell you about your diet?"
"Can you tell me about your job responsibilities in your previous position?"
"How did you become interested in this position?"

Closed questions are more restrictive, that is, they limit answers. Some closed questions are more limiting than others. Examples are:

"Who cooks the meals at home?"
"Can you tell me about any snacks you eat?"
"What skills do you have that are important for this job?"

Closed questions give the interviewer more control, require less effort from the interviewee, and are less time-consuming. Disadvantages include the inhibition of communication, which might result if the interviewer shows little interest in the answers, taking more questions to obtain the same information, and getting answers that may not reveal why the respondent feels as he does.

Primary and Secondary Questions. Questions may also be classified as primary or secondary. Primary questions introduce new topics or areas. The following are examples.

*"Now that we have discussed your most recent position, can you tell me about
    your former job with Smith & Co.?"*
*"Now that we have discussed the food you eat at home, tell me about what
    you eat in restaurants."*

Note that referring to what was just said shows that one has been
listening.

Secondary questions attempt to obtain further information or explanation that primary questions have failed to elicit; they may be
referred to as "follow-up" questions. Interviewees may have given
an inadequate response for many reasons, including poor memory,
misunderstanding of the question or amount of detail desired, and
the feeling that the question is too personal or irrelevant, or that
the professional would not understand the response. Specific follow-
up questions, such as the following, may be asked:

"How much orange juice do you drink?"
"What do you use in your coffee?"
"In your previous position, how many people did you supervise?"

Neutral and Leading Questions. Neutral questions are preferred
to leading questions. Leading questions direct the respondent to
one answer in preference to others, an effect that may be unintentional on the part of the interviewer. Leading questions reveal the
bias of the interviewer, which he himself may not recognize. Examples are:

"You eat breakfast, don't you?" "Yes, of course."
"You aren't going to eat desserts anymore, are you?" "No."
"What do you eat for breakfast?" "An egg and toast."

Two of these questions assume that the client consumes breakfast, and in these instances, the client will probably answer as he
feels he is expected to, even if he usually omits the meal. The client
may change his answers on the basis of nonverbal appearances in
the dietitian of surprise, disgust, dislike, or disagreement with what
the client is saying. To receive uninhibited responses from the client,
the interviewer should try to avoid these appearances.

The dietitian's language and wording must be understood by the
client if successful communication is to take place. One does not
need to impress people with medical and dietetic vocabulary. Complex terminology should be avoided, or used sparingly, and only
when one is sure that the client understands. The following may be
misunderstood:

*"People with the type of hyperlipidemia you have should avoid eating foods
    containing saturated fatty acids and emphasize polyunsaturates instead."*

When the interviewer senses that too many questions are being
asked and that the respondent may be developing a "feeling of
interrogation," he may introduce some questions as a statement or
directive.[1] For example, "How has your diet been going?" may be

changed to "I'd be interested in hearing how your diet has been going." "How did you become interested in this position?" may be changed to "I'd be interested in some of the reasons you decided to apply for this position." This makes the interview more conversational.

Questions should be asked one at a time, and the interviewer should concentrate on listening carefully to the answers rather than thinking ahead to the next question to be asked. Further discussion of questions is found in Chapter 4.

Sequence of Questions. Questions are often arranged in a "funnel" sequence.[9] A funnel sequence begins with broad, open questions and proceeds to more restrictive ones, for example:

> *"Tell me about the food you eat during the day."*
> *"What do you have for snacks between meals?"*
> *"We haven't discussed alcoholic beverages—what about them?"*

Beginning with open-ended questions poses the least threat to the client and induces him to talk. The person then volunteers much information, making it necessary to ask fewer questions. At times, an inverted funnel sequence may be preferable. In preemployment interviews, for example, applicants may feel more comfortable dealing with a specific question than with a broad, open one, such as "Tell me about yourself," when they are apprehensive and unsure of what to say or what the interviewer expects.

In taking a diet history, questions or statements starting with "What" or "Tell me about" elicit better responses than those starting with "Do you . . . ?" Examples include the following:

> *"I'd like to get some background about your daily food intake starting with when your arise in the morning. Tell me about the first meal or food you eat during the day—what you eat, and in what amounts."*
> *"Tell me about the next meal or food you eat. What would it be like?"*
> *"Now that we have discussed your meals, can you tell me about coffee breaks or the types of snacks you eat between meals and the times of day you eat them?"*
> *"We haven't talked about beverages. What about beer, wine, and alcohol?"*

These questions or statements allow the person to tell his story in his own way.

Questions that do not require a complete answer or that may be answered with one word or with "Yes" or "No" are less productive, such as the following:

> *"Do you eat breakfast?" "Yes."*
> *"Do you drink orange juice?" "Yes."*
> *"Do you eat cereal for breakfast?" "No."*
> *"Do you like milk?" "No."*
> *"How often do you eat meat?" "Once a day."*

A series of short, sequential, dead-end questions from the professional's list of information to be gathered prevents the person from telling his story in his own way, and information may be omitted as a result.

In the follow-up visits, opening questions should be broad to allow the client to determine the focus of the interview. Examples are "Tell me how the diet is going" and "What progress have you made since we last talked?" The dietitian should begin discussion with whatever is of current concern to the patient. For opening questions, the dietitian should also refer to his records regarding the client and his problems, and other information.

Bernstein recommends avoiding questions beginning with "Why."[7] While asking "why" may seek information, it may also indicate disapproval or mistrust and appear to ask for justification or explanation, for example:

> *"Why don't you follow your diet?"*
> *"Why don't you eat breakfast?"*
> *"Why did you resign from your job?"*

The client may react defensively or explain his behavior in a manner he believes is acceptable to the dietitian.

> *"Because I don't understand my diet."*
> *"I'll start eating breakfast tomorrow if you think I should."*
> *"Because there was no chance for advancement."*

If threatened by a "why" question and unwilling to reveal the answer, the individual may answer in an evasive manner, in which case nothing is gained.

Responses. In the verbal interaction of medical interviews, Bernstein maintains that interviewer responses may be divided into five categories: (1) evaluation, (2) hostility, (3) reassurance, (4) probing, and (5) understanding.[7] A sixth response, confrontation, should be used only by an experienced interviewer. In the discussion of each type, responses to the following statement by a client are compared: "I haven't lost any weight this week. I ate just a few cookies. The diet doesn't work."

Evaluation. In the evaluative response, the interviewer makes a judgment about the person's feelings or responses or implies how the person ought to feel. The evaluative response leads to the offering of advice by the professional for the solution of the client's problem. An example is "I suggest that you stop buying those cookies." Note that the evaluative response leads to the giving of advice, not information. Little attempt is made to understand the psychological needs of the patient or the reason that the cookies were eaten. The recipient of the advice has the choice of following it or not. At times, advice is ignored as a means of maintaining one's independence.

Hostility. In the hostile response, the professional's anger is uncontrolled, and the response may lead to antagonism or humiliation of the client. The following response is an example: "You're not acting very mature. I've told you before to avoid all sweets and desserts if you want to lose weight." The hostile response may lead the client to a reply that retaliates: "How would you know about dieting? Look how thin you are." A vicious cycle of angry, hostile responses results, destroying the professional/client relationship. The fact that the client is anxious about the inability to follow the diet has been ignored by the professional. The dietitian who is frustrated by the client who is not following the diet should avoid responding with anger.

Reassurance. With a reassuring response, the client is prevented from working through his feelings since the interviewer suggests that there is nothing to worry about. Frequently, a client's expressions of anxiety are followed by the dietitian's reassuring response that things will improve and that the person should not worry, as illustrated by the following: "Don't worry about it. It takes time to adjust to new eating patterns. You'll do better next week." This response suggests that the problem does not exist, or that the professional does not want to discuss it. Such responses make it difficult to solve the client's problem or to discuss it further. Admission of failure may have been difficult for the client, but it indicated a desire to discuss the problem.

Probing. The probing response is an attempt to gain additional information. It implies that the person should give more information so that the professional can assist in solving the problem. "So you think the diet doesn't work; I wonder if you could tell me a little more about that." This helps the person to tell his story, and further information can be obtained.

There are several probing techniques, which may be used to facilitate better interviewee responses in addition to secondary or follow-up questions. They should be nonthreatening and nonjudgmental. A brief silence may be effective, as may repetition of the last phrase spoken by the client or a summary sentence. Closing probes may elicit important additional information. Probing further in the case of superficial and vague responses, as well as probing for feelings about events, is suggested in the following paragraphs.

When a more detailed response is desired in the case of superficial answers, the following may be asked:

"Can you tell me more about that?"
"What do you do next?"
"Please explain a little more about ...."
"Anything else?"

To obtain clarification when the answer is vague, one may respond:

"Could you clarify for me what you meant by ...?"
"I don't think I quite understand ...."

Paraphrasing is another technique to ensure that the information is clear and correct. By repeating, summarizing, or rewording what was said, the interviewer shows that he is trying to understand.

When the person seems hesitant to go on, the interviewer may remain silent, pausing for the respondent to gather his thoughts and continue. The professional should appear attentive, with perhaps a thoughtful or expectant look, but should avoid eye contact for the moment. While the inexperienced interviewer may find silence un-comfortable and embarrassing and push on too quickly, a more experienced interviewer realizes that too hasty a response may cause part of the story to remain untold or change what is disclosed. If the interviewee does not go on within 30 to 60 seconds, however, he may perceive the silence as disinterest or disapproval; the inter-viewer should commence before that impression can occur.

A technique useful in breaking a silence is to repeat or echo the last phrase or sentence the person has said, raising the tone of voice to a question. For example:

> *"I follow my diet except when I eat out."*
> *"Except when you eat out?"*

Repetition, however, should not be overdone, or it can have a parrot-like effect. If this is noticed by the respondent, it will inhibit con-versation.

A summary sentence stated as a question also elicits further elab-oration. For example:

> *"You say you already know the exchange system for diabetic diets?"*
> *"You think this company is the one you want to work for?"*

Other probes are:

> *"Go on."*
> *"I see."*
> *"I understand. Please continue."*
> *"Uh huh."*
> *"Hmmmm."*
> *"And next?"*
> *"Oh?"* or *"Oh!"*
> *"Really?"*
> *"Very good!"*
> *"That's interesting!"*

"I see," "I understand," and "that's interesting" may give a feeling of acceptance and encourage conversation or elaboration of a point of view. "Very good" gives the person a pat on the back, and is another kind of acceptance comment. Nonverbal probes include giving a quizzical look, leaning forward in the chair, and nodding the head.

Understanding. In the understanding response the interviewer tries to understand the person's message and re-create it within his own frame of reference. People have more rapport with those who try to understand them, and this may lead to more cooperation on the part of the client. "You are feeling concerned because you haven't lost any weight, and you are wondering if it was something you ate, or a problem with the diet." The understanding response assists the person to clarify what was stated. The person also feels accepted even if his behavior has not been perfect. The client will feel safe in expressing his sentiments and exploring them further. The client who believes that the professional is an understanding person may cooperate more fully in the interview.

Note that the professional should focus on the client's feelings and attitudes, rather than only on the content of what is being said. In the example given, the client may be expressing his feelings of disappointment with the diet, his dissatisfaction with lack of progress in weight loss, his frustration about changing eating habits, or his fear of the dietitian's response to the fact that no weight has been lost. The understanding response should be most helpful in assisting the client to recognize problems and to devise his own solutions. He may progress from initial negative feelings to more neutral ones and finally to more positive attitudes and solutions. Expressions of sincere sympathy may assist in building bridges in personal relationships, especially in response to information about death, prolonged illness, discomfort, or other problems. A quick response may be "Oh, my!" or "I'm very sorry to hear that."

It is necessary to differentiate and understand both the content of a message and the feelings. To determine the content, one may ask oneself, "What is this person telling me or thinking?" In identifying feelings, ask, "What is this person feeling, and why is he feeling that way?" As in the previous example, the answer may be inserted into a format such as "He feels ... because...." One may use such a sentence to paraphrase the person's statement to verify one's understanding. Although one may have an incorrect impression, such as feeling that a person is bored when the person actually is fatigued, the interviewee will usually provide the correct interpretation, thereby furthering the interviewer's understanding; this process demonstrates that one is trying to understand.

Interviewee responses that suggest feelings about an event may provide an important key to understanding the person's behavior. How the patient or client feels about his lifestyle, his diet, or his health is critical to dietary adherence. Food behaviors may be influenced by psychological, cultural, and environmental variables that are important to understand. Job applicants may also express feelings about previous work experience, relationships with superiors and subordinates, and activities and interests. Preceding a statement with "I think," "I feel," or "I believe" gives a signal that the statement

expresses opinions, beliefs, attitudes, and values. Appropriate follow-up probes may be the following:

> *"Can you explain more about your feelings?"*
> *"What do YOU think about that?"*
> *"What do you think causes that?"*

Confrontation. Confrontation is an authority-laden response in
which the interviewer verbally calls to the person's attention some
startling aspect of verbal or nonverbal behavior that he may not have
recognized, for example:

> *"You seem to have a lot of difficulty following your diet."*
> *"It sounds like you didn't get along well with your previous supervisor."*

This response challenges the person to recognize and cope psychologically with some aspect of behavior that is self-defeating, or
to examine the consequences of some behavior. Confrontation
should not be used by an inexperienced interviewer or when good
rapport and a supportive atmosphere are missing. Otherwise, such
responses can become threatening or appear punitive, and will inhibit conversation.[8,11]

During the interview, one can examine not only what the person
says, but also what he does not say. Are there gaps in the information
that the interviewer should try to fill? One should also note nonverbal
behaviors, such as tension, inability to maintain eye contact, hand
movements, fidgeting, and facial expressions of discomfort, nervousness, anger, or lack of understanding. The nonverbal behaviors
may be inconsistent with the verbal message, or may add to it.

While the interviewer should adjust the pace of the interview to
that of the respondent, he is also responsible for the direction of
the interview. When the topics for discussion are inappropriate, the
skilled interviewer brings the conversation back to appropriate areas.
The patient talking about his wife or his children, for example, must
be brought gently back to the diet history. A job applicant discussing
a recent visit to Spain must be brought back to relevant topics.
People who are especially talkative may ramble frequently, requiring
more leadership on the part of the interviewer. In these cases, re-
stating or emphasizing the last thing said that was pertinent to the
interview, and asking a related question, may be helpful.

Closing

The third part or closing of the interview takes the shortest amount
of time, but should not be rushed or taken lightly. A word of appreciation sincerely expressed, such as thanking the person for his
time and cooperation, is a common closing. Another suggestion is
to review the purpose of the interview and declare its completion.
One may ask if the interviewee has any questions he would like to

ask or any other comments he wants to make, which may elicit important new information for which adequate time should be available. The time, place, and purpose of future contacts should be mentioned. To a hospitalized patient, the dietitian may say, "I'll stop by to see you tomorrow to discuss your diet with you." With a client, arrangements for a future appointment may be made. To make sure that each has understood the other, plans may be paraphrased.

As a courtesy to job applicants, the dietitian should tell them approximately when the employment decision will be made and how they will be contacted if selected, for example, "If selected, you'll hear from us in about a week by telephone." For those not selected, a letter may be sent thanking them for their applications and interest in the company and telling them that the position has been filled. This letter is a public relations effort that can be handled by the personnel department. The applicant who hears nothing after an interview may react negatively or telephone again for information. One may signal the close of the interview by breaking eye contact, placing hands on the arms of the chair, standing up, offering to shake hands, smiling, and waving goodbye.

Interviewing is a skill, and as with other skills, it takes practice to develop. The inexperienced interviewer needs to plan in writing what topics need to be covered and in what sequence. Various types of questions can be prepared in advance in an appropriate sequence for the three parts of the interview. Physical surroundings and freedom from interruption should be planned. These conditions put the professional in a better position to concentrate on the interviewee and on the process of developing rapport, noting the verbal and nonverbal responses and providing understanding responses with empathy. The interview session should be followed by a self-evaluation to determine areas that went well, as well as those that could be improved for the next interview.

SUGGESTED ACTIVITIES

1. Watch an interview on television noting the parts of the interview, techniques used, and verbal and nonverbal responses. Use the evaluation form in Appendix D, if appropriate.

2. Plan an interview guide specifying content and sequence. Write examples of various kinds of questions, such as open and closed, primary and secondary, neutral and leading.

3. Divide into groups of two with each person interviewing the other in turn. When this is completed, use the evaluation form in Appendix D to complete an evaluation. If three people are available, the third may serve as evaluator.

4. Make an audiotape of a simulated or actual interview, if participants' permission is granted. Complete an evaluation.

5. Make a videotape of a simulated or actual interview, if participants' permission is granted. This will show nonverbal behaviors as well as any personal idiosyncrasies. Complete an evaluation.

REFERENCES

1. Morgan, J., and Cogger, J.: The Interviewer's Manual. 2nd ed. New York, Drake Beam Morin, 1980.
2. Chruden, H.J., and Sherman, A.W.: Managing Human Resources. 7th ed. Cincinnati, South-Western Pub. Co., 1984.
3. Mathis, R.L., and Jackson, J.H.: Personnel: Human Resource Management. 4th ed. St. Paul, West Pub. Co., 1985.
4. Olson, R.: Managing the Interview. New York, John Wiley and Sons, 1980.
5. Jasmund, J.M.: The Diet History: A Tool and A Process. East Lansing, Michigan State University Press, 1981.
6. Mason, M., Wenberg, B.G., and Welsch, P.K.: The Dynamics of Clinical Dietetics. 2nd ed. New York, John Wiley and Sons, 1982.
7. Bernstein, L., and Bernstein, R.S.: Interviewing: A Guide for Health Professionals. 3rd ed. New York, Appleton-Century-Crofts, 1980.
8. Wiese, H.J.C.: The Diet Interview: A How-To Guide. ACS 8. Chicago, American Dietetic Assoc., 1984.
9. Stewart, C.J., and Cash, W.B.: Interviewing: Principles and Practices. 4th ed. Dubuque, IA, Wm. C. Brown, 1985.
10. Lozez, F.: Personnel Interviewing. 2nd ed. New York, McGraw-Hill, 1975.
11. Engen, H., Iasiello-Vailas, L., and Smith, K.: Confrontation: A new dimension in nutritional counseling. J. Am. Diet. Assoc., *83*:34, 1983.

4

Counseling

In recent years, the profession of dietetics has experienced profound changes as the scope of practice has broadened. As the roles and responsibilities of dietitians have changed, so has the need for knowledge and skills in different subjects. According to the 1984 Study Commission on Dietetics, one area of educational preparation of dietitians that needs greater emphasis is communication skills.[1] Role delineation studies conducted by the American Dietetic Association in the areas of clinical dietetics, community dietetics, and food service systems management confirmed the need for dietitians to be knowledgeable of the process of communication in general, and the techniques of counseling in particular.[2-4]

Today a considerable portion of the dietitian's time may be spent counseling. For a professional member of the health care team in clinical practice, counseling skills are applied in nutrition counseling, and for an administrative dietitian, they are utilized in counseling staff. Counseling can be defined as a process that assists an individual in learning about himself, his environment, and methods of handling his roles and relationships. It involves problem solving, identifying goals, and change. Counselors assist individuals with the decision-making process, resolving interpersonal concerns, and helping them to learn new ways of dealing with and adjusting to life situations.

This chapter presents an overview of the counseling process as it applies to dietitians. Counseling may be considered a four-stage process, with the first stage involving the development of a trusting, helping relationship between counselor and counselee, and the next three stages concentrated on problem solving. In addition, approaches to counseling, classified as either nondirective or directive, are compared. The nondirective or "client-centered" approach originated by Carl Rogers is described and applied to the nutritional counseling of clients and patients. Guidelines for directive counseling are also provided and applied to the counseling of subordinate staff regarding job-related problems.

ROGERIAN CLIENT-CENTERED COUNSELING

The nondirective approach to counseling is often called "client-centered" and is best represented by the writing of its originator, Carl Ransom Rogers (1902—). Dr. Rogers' theory was first presented in his book *Counseling and Psychotherapy* (1942), and was further developed in his later books.[5-6] Although the theory is constantly developing, changing with experience and research, there seems to have been no basic change in its assumptions. The theory is one of the more detailed, integrated, and consistent theories currently existing and has led to, and is supported by, a greater amount of research then any other approach to counseling.[7] Rather than providing a complete description of the theory, the following discussion is intended to acquaint the reader with some of its more salient assumptions, particularly, those related to the counseling techniques described later in this chapter.

Contrary to the common concept that man is by nature irrational, unsocialized, and destructive of himself and others, a basic assumption in the client-centered point of view is that man is basically rational, socialized, and realistic. Each individual, if his needs for positive regard from others and for positive self-regard are satisfied, possesses an inherent tendency toward realizing his potential for growth and self-actualization. Counseling releases the potentials and capacities of the individual.

One of the most important characteristics of this theory is the relationship it suggests between the counselor and the client. The underlying assumption is that the client cannot be helped simply by listening to the knowledge the counselor possesses or to the counselor's explanation of the client's personality or behavior. Prescribing "cures" and corrective behavior are seen as being of little lasting value. The relationship that is most helpful to the client, that enables him to discover within himself the capacity to use the relationship to change and grow, is not a cognitive, intellectual one. Rogers states: "I believe the quality of my encounter is more important in the long run than is my scholarly knowledge, my professional training, my counseling orientation, the techniques I use in the interview."[8] There are four specific characteristics that Rogers suggests the counselor possess for the therapy relationship: acceptance, congruence, understanding, and the ability to communicate these to the client.

The counselor needs to be accepting of the client as an individual, as he is, with his good and bad points, his conflicts and inconsistencies. Only after the client is convinced that he is accepted unconditionally and nonjudgmentally can he begin to trust the counselor.

The ideal counselor is characterized by congruence within the counseling relationship. He is unified, integrated, and consistent, with no contradictions between what he is and what he says. The counselor is able to express outwardly to his client what he is feeling within himself. His verbal and nonverbal behaviors are consistent.

The counselor must experience an accurate, empathic understanding of the client's world as seen from the inside, sensing the client's world as if it were his own, but without losing the "as if" quality. This empathy is essential to nondirective therapy. The understanding enables the client to explore freely and deeply, and develop a better comprehension of himself.

It is of no value for the counselor to be accepting, congruent, and understanding if the client does not perceive or experience this. The acceptance, congruence, and understanding need to be communicated to the client verbally and nonverbally. Rogers is definite in his belief that these not be "techniques," but a genuine and spontaneous expression of the counselor's inner attitudes.[7]

If the counselor has these characteristics and attitudes and is able to communicate them to his client, then a relationship develops that is experienced by the client as safe, secure, free from threat, and supportive. The counselor is perceived as dependable, trustworthy, and consistent. This is a relationship in which change can occur.

Understanding One's Need to Be a Counselor. Because one's own needs for being a counselor affect the helping interactions, it is essential that counselors become aware of their own motivations in choosing to help others. Generally these include doing good, having contact with people, earning a living, and fulfilling a personal commitment. Often, however, there may be deeper motivations as well. Helping satisfies basic needs; it may provide a salary, but it also satisfies psychological needs. For example, counselors may become involved in helping others to resolve problems or to satisfy personal needs for power, prestige, and the dependency of others. A counselor's needs do affect the process of helping others. For example, a counselor with a strong need to be needed might extend a helping relationship unnecessarily to gratify the need. A counselor with a need for power may take too much control over the counselee's situation or give too much advice. A counselor's need to be seen as competent can also interfere with the process of helping. If he tends to take personal responsibility for his counselees' successes and failures, he will become upset when counselees do not change. Counseling is influenced by the counselor's personal needs and motivations; therefore, it is crucial that the counselor understands these needs prior to engaging in counseling to ensure that they do not interfere with his efforts to help.[9]

COUNSELING AS A FOUR-STAGE PROCESS

In accordance with the theoretical assumptions of nondirective counseling, many counselors, trainers, educators, and theoreticians consider counseling to be a four-stage process, with the first stage involving the development of rapport, empathy, and a trusting relationship, and the three subsequent stages involving the implementation of specific behavioral change strategies and techniques directed at the client's problem. Counseling deals simultaneously with both content and feelings. Trained counselors realize that only after the client's underlying feelings have been exposed and talked about can the content behind those feelings be discussed. Each stage requires special counseling skills that may have a particular utility and relevance at that stage. A model of the helping process, developed by Dennis Kinlaw,[10] is shown in Figure 4-1.

The first stage, *involving,* may be initiated by either the client or the counselor, but the goals of this stage remain the same—to give the client clear expectations of the counseling process and a level of comfort and trust enabling him to interact authentically and effectively with the counselor. The counselor's sincere concern and caring must be established during this stage or the remainder of the counseling process is likely to be ineffective. Concern and caring are often expressed in ways other than words. The old adage is valid: actions speak louder than words. If the counselor seems uninterested, the counselee is likely to feel uncomfortable and confused. Attentive nonverbal behavior allows one to infer caring and concern and creates the impression that the counselor is capable and effective. Counselors need to be conscious of eye contact, body posture, hand and arm movements, facial expressions, and vocal quality because these are the signals by which clients infer the degree of attentiveness, caring, and concern. A counselor's words can make a difference, however. They can encourage the counselee to discuss a concern with greater openness or they can limit the counselee's disclosures. One must learn a new set of verbal responses, each of which is useful for a specific purpose.

Stages II, III, and IV relate more specifically to the recognition and initiation of specific behavior-change strategies. Stage II, *exploring,* can begin once trust has been established. The goal is to discuss the nature of the specific problem in concrete rather than vague terms. The counselor's role is to encourage the counselee to enlarge on all issues and provide details related to the problem. He does this through the use of the numerous helping skills included in the helping-process model. In stage III, *resolving,* the counselee's goal is to begin planning some actions to resolve the problem. The counselor, mostly through the use of questions, attempts to collaborate, suggest alternatives, and serve as a resource to the counselee. The final stage, *concluding,* is intended to verify for the counselee the plan for subsequent actions. The counselor may reinforce the proposed actions of the counselee, but his primary task is to make

Helping-Process Model

Process Stages	Goals for the Helpee	Helper Roles	Helping Skills
I: Involving	Clear expectations Comfort Trust	*Responder:* Helper responds to initiative taken by helpee. *Initiator:* Helper takes initiative.	*Inviting:* Encouraging helpee to begin or continue *Acknowledging:* Making comments such as "yes," "uh-huh," "okay," and so forth *Giving negative feedback:* Giving feedback regarding a performance-related problem (supervisor to subordinate) *Offering assistance:* Indicating desire to help *Attending:* Using verbal and nonverbal behaviors to focus on helpee and using senses to detect helpee's entire message *Avoiding disrespect:* Avoiding responses that communicate judgment, disregard helpee's feelings and opinions, and so forth *Being genuine:* Being oneself; avoiding "role" behaviors
II: Exploring	Information Awareness Understanding Insight Discussion of problem in concrete terms	*Encourager/stimulator:* Helper's responses enlarge data surrounding problem; helper clarifies perceptions.	*Skills from previous stage as appropriate* *Reflecting:* Playing back feelings and content of helpee's comments *Identifying:* Indicating that helper has had similar experience or feeling *Discussing the helping transaction:* Exploring problems arising from transaction itself *Searching:* Using questions or statements that are relevant and nonthreatening *Testing:* Clarifying and summarizing helper's own understanding *Confronting:* Presenting helpee with possible inconsistencies, avoidances, missed connections, and so forth
III: Resolving	Problem definition Problem ownership Action planning	*Collaborator:* Helper treats problem definitively, suggests alternatives, and serves as a resource.	*Skills from previous stages as appropriate* *Problem stating:* Testing with possible statements of problem *Identifying resources:* Sharing leads, insights, interpretations, and information with helpee *Action planning:* Collaborating with helpee to develop change plans
IV: Concluding	Optimism Direction	*Concluder:* Helper refocuses on purpose of conversation; reinforces results; and resists introduction of new, evocative material.	*Skills from previous stages as appropriate* *Reinforcing:* Identifying strengths, gains, and insights; restating action plans and expectations *Summarizing:* Listing explicit issues discussed, actions planned, and so forth *Appreciating:* Commenting on helpee's cooperation, use of time, and so forth

Fig. 4-1. Helping model. (From Kinlaw, D.: Helping Skills for Human Resource Development: A Facilitator's Package. San Diego, CA, University Associates, Inc., 1981. Used with permission.)

certain that both he and the counselee agree on what has occurred during the session and on all subsequent actions that are to take place.

DIRECTIVE AND NONDIRECTIVE COUNSELING

The remainder of this chapter focuses on the general applications of directive and nondirective counseling strategies as they might be used in nutritional counseling and in employee counseling. Counselees perceive the two counseling strategies differently, and their responses to the two strategies differ. Directive counseling tends to be most appropriate when the counselor is aware of the problem and/or is concerned about the behavior of the counselee but the counselee is unaware of the problem or is avoiding acknowledging it. Nondirective counseling tends to be most appropriate when the counselee has insight and calls on the counselor to assist in the problem solving.

In the first instance, directive counseling, the counselor initiates discussion or summons the counselee. In the second instance, nondirective counseling, the counselee is aware of the problem and seeks help from the counselor. Counselees tend to be far more likely to become defensive and resist problem solving under the conditions of directive counseling. For this reason, counselors employing the method need to be especially sensitive to all verbal and nonverbal behavior, being supportive while attempting to explore the problem areas.

Directive counseling probably occurs most often in the manager/subordinate relationship rather than in the dietitian/client relationship. In general, directive counseling techniques are used to expose poor employee performance when the employee is unaware or unwilling to expose it himself. Nondirective counseling is ordinarily the preferred counseling method when dealing with clients who need to plan and set wellness goals or with employees who have sought out the help of their manager or supervisor. Frequently, counselors employ a combination of both methods, but for discussion purposes, each is described separately. Nondirective counseling is described first.

Applications of Nondirective Counseling

Involving Stage. When a client seeks out a dietitian directly, or when a dietitian has been recommended by a physician, the dietitian should first allow the client to expose his own concerns fully before giving any advice. The dietitian may be rushed, and anxious to prescribe a diet regimen, but the regimen is likely to be ignored unless the patient himself has participated in the plan and has developed trust and a sense of confidence in the dietitian. An earlier chapter has elaborated on the necessity for clients to vent all of their concerns so that they are mentally receptive to listening. It is the nondirective counselor's responsibility to encourage "venting." Sometimes patients are ill at ease with professional helpers and hesitate to talk. The dietitian may need to learn to tolerate some silence and to be reassuring and supportive when he attempts to induce the client to reveal underlying concerns.

Because underlying problems are frequently emotional rather than logical and are not likely to be revealed until the counselee trusts the counselor, the counselor's learning to respond without giving advice or passing judgment is essential. This response is especially important in the case of the administrative dietitian working with a staff member. An employee's reasons for occasional abruptness with patients or apparent lack of interest in his job may be due to some illogical prejudice rather than laziness. He may be aware of the problem and may want to correct it, but before he reveals the underlying cause, he will certainly want assurance that he will not be humiliated or embarrassed for doing so. An employee who is frequently late to work because of family problems, for example, may have underlying emotional and illogical explanations for his behavior. Revealing these reasons to a counselor usually occurs, if it occurs at all, only after less honest but more logical reasons have been presented and the counselee is confident he can be honest without being belittled.

Exploring Stage. There is little value in the counselor's making recommendations until he has first fully understood the client's perspective and gained the client's trust. The client himself becomes far more receptive to hearing the counselor's advice when he is certain that he has said all he wants to say and that his words have been understood. During the exploring stage, the dietitian attempts to provide insight for the counselee by clarifying perceptions and attempting to discuss the problems in concrete terms.

In reality, not all clients, whether patients or subordinates, are articulate and able to express themselves. Although they may want to express themselves, they may have a difficult time exposing their concerns. The counselor can offer assistance by asking questions that stimulate full explanations. Two kinds of questions used in counseling are "open-ended questions" and "closed-ended questions." Understanding the distinction between the two is important because each tends to elicit a different response from the counselee. The use of directives or "encouragers" and active listening are helpful.

Closed-Ended Questions. Closed-ended questions are designed to be answered by brief responses (often by one or two words, or by "yes" or "no"). They are good for eliciting specific data quickly. Examples include questions such as "When did you notice you were gaining excess weight?" or "How many times have you asked to leave early in the past two weeks?" One of the limitations of closed-ended questions is that they do not promote any explanation or elaboration on the question asked and are controlled totally by the questioner. Also, they tend to be characterized by the concepts "who," "where," or "when," or they are statements turned into questions. Additional examples include "Who is responsible for your department's high turnover?" "Where do you tend to do most of your eating?" and "When do you find yourself craving sweets most?"

Open-Ended Questions. Open-ended questions are designed to encourage longer answers. They are good for eliciting responses in the other's own words, and for encouraging the other to enlarge on an idea and to reveal all concerns. The major difficulty with open-ended questions is that they take longer to answer and can be frustrating when specific data are needed and time pressures are present. They tend to be characterized by the words "how," "what," and "why." "How did you initially try to lose weight on your own?" "What sorts of treatments have you tried in the past?" and "Why do you want to be a size three?" are examples of open-ended questions.

The skill of asking specific closed-ended questions when a short and concise direct answer is desired and open-ended questions when a fuller and more subjective answer is desired is not natural for most people. The explanation and examples given previously may make it seem simple. It is not! Developing this ability takes practice, and both students and professionals wishing to increase their competence in question formation should make a conscious effort to practice it whenever possible. Over time, the skills become automatic and one begins to frame questions easily, either to elicit specific answers or to allow the counselee to move the discussion subjectively into other areas.

Use of Directives. There will be times when even open-ended questions fail to lead the client to expand on an idea or give additional information. The response may be a simple shrug of the shoulders, or "I don't know" or "I don't remember." When this occurs, there is an additional verbal response possible from the counselor that is often effective. It is called a "directive." A directive involves the use of a command rather than a question. It should not, of course, sound like a command and put the client on the defensive, but when delivered in a gentle, supportive manner, directives often do what open-ended questions cannot do with hesitant clients—get them to talk more. Examples of directives include comments such as "Talk more about ..."; "I want to know what you think of ..."; "Tell me your ideas on ..."; "Expand on your thoughts regarding. ..."

Use of Encouragers. In addition to the use of open-ended questions, closed-ended questions, and directives, counselors need to develop their ability to use nonverbal "encouragers." Encouragers are sometimes verbal utterances such as "Yes, yes," "Ah ha," or "Hmmmm," or some other sound that indicates to the client that the counselor is listening and comprehending. These utterances should be accompanied by such nonverbal signs as nodding the head, leaning forward toward the client, and making other facial expressions that suggest interest, understanding, and the desire for the client to go on speaking. Frequently, the best way to get the client to talk more is for the counselor to remain silent when the client stops talking. After a few moments of silence without the counselor filling in the awkward moments, the client is apt to go on talking if he has more to add.

Active Listening. It has been mentioned that prior to the counselor's asking questions, probing into specific areas, giving advice, passing judgment on the rightness or wrongness of the client's behavior, or disclosing his own experiences, he must first be certain that he has understood the problems as the client intends. This is done through the use of active listening—paraphrasing and responding empathically. After the counselor has understood the original problem to the counselee's satisfaction, and at each subsequent stage in the counseling process, the counselor needs to repeat the verification process through paraphrase and empathic responses. Communicators need to remember that they don't know what they don't know. Everyone is subject unconsciously to selective perception and communication distortion. For that reason, a summary paraphrase and an empathic reaction are appropriate at each stage in the counseling process. Besides verifying for the counselor that he is understanding the counselee as intended, the paraphrase summary often provides real insight for the counselee. Just hearing the same comments in another person's words can help the counselee to see new possibilities and to have new insight.

The underlying principle governing the use of nondirective counseling is that when the client seeks help, he is often the person in the best position to solve his problem and to suggest corrective behavior. The job of the counselor is to help the counselee to understand his problem more clearly and, in nutritional counseling, to make him aware of alternatives available for solving the problem. In nondirective counseling, the technique for doing this is called "mirroring." The counselor "mirrors" or reflects back to the counselee what he has said. When this is done in a supportive manner, without the subjective values and judgments of the counselor added, the process tends to stimulate creative thinking and understanding in the counselee. Part of the "supportive manner" for counselors includes the ability to make responses without sounding clinical. Comments such as "What I hear you saying is . . ." or "Run that past me again" may be interpreted as sounding clinical and officious. It is more supportive to say, "I just want to be sure I'm understanding. Is this what you are saying . . .?"

Resolving Stage. Once the total problem has been explored and understood, the counselor and counselee can move on to examine the criteria for solving the problem, which form the framework for any solution. The specific purpose of this stage is to assist the counselee in setting goals and identifying resources for resolving the problem. As mentioned earlier, all stages of the process are primarily interrogative for the counselor. He moves through the stages by asking questions, not by judging. He might say to someone with high blood pressure and a problem of eating too many high-sodium foods, for example, "What are some low-sodium snacks that could be substituted for potato chips?" To someone whose problem is eating too many high-calorie desserts and whose goal is to lose weight, he might ask about the possibility of selecting fruit for dessert for the next seven days or the possibility of purchasing lower-fat meats for the next week.

Throughout the process, discipline is required of the counselor. Often, he will be tempted to say, "Can't you see, this is what you need to do!" or "This is what you must do." The problem in being prescriptive, that is, telling the counselee what he must do to solve his problem, is that the solutions arrived at in that manner are not really the counselee's; they are the counselor's. A solution that a person has struggled to form himself is more likely to work than one "given" to him by another person. If the solution prescribed by the counselor does not work, the counselee can always say, "I told you so," or "You didn't really understand what I meant." Also, when counselors dictate solutions to counselees, they are likely to receive the response, "Yes, but . . ." from the counselee. The counselee tends to rationalize a reason for rejecting whatever the counselor prescribes. Although the alternative method takes longer and requires more discipline, the counselor will be more effective in the nondirective process if he coaches the counselee to make all decisions himself, whenever possible.

After the criteria for a solution are made clear, the counselor needs to help the counselee formulate several alternative solutions. This process may take time, discipline, and patience. Frequently, one solution is obvious, while other possible solutions remain in the client's unconscious. A counselor with discipline and patience can bring other potential solutions to the consciousness of his client by helping him to focus on other possibilities and not allowing him to rush off on refining the single first alternative. Some open-ended questions useful at this stage are "What solutions have you tried already?" "What are some things that might help?" "Are there other possibilities you haven't yet thought of?" Allowing time for silent reflection on the part of the counselee during this process is critical.

After several alternatives have been listed, the counselor may add some of his own. As the nutrition expert, the dietitian has knowledge and insight to suggest alternatives unknown to the client. It is important, however, to add additional suggestions in a way that leaves the counselee free to reject any and all. The difference between "Here is one thing you might consider" and "Here is what you need to do" is that if the former is accepted as the solution, the counselee considers it his own idea and will be committed to making it work; if the latter is selected, the counselee considers it the counselor's idea and is less committed to making it work.

There will also be times when the alternative selected by the counselee is obviously a poor choice. Here the counselor may be tempted to say, "Can't you see what a poor solution that is?" or even worse, "That is a terrible idea." Rather than pass negative judgments, the counselor would do better to assist the counselee in understanding the weaknesses in the solution. This can be done through the use of open-ended questions that will foster the counselee's involvement in evaluating the solution himself. The counselor might ask, for example, "What would happen if you tried that? Would the situation get better or worse?" In this way, the counselee, not the counselor, is rejecting the solution.

Concluding Stage. It is possible for a client, whether employee or patient, to go through the entire process previously described and not internalize the agreed upon solution and action plan. Because most people are not accustomed to being counseled, and because of the status distinction between the counselor and counselee, the counselee may feel a heightened anxiety, which causes him to distort meanings and block clear understanding. He may be agreeing and nodding understanding when, in fact, his own nervousness is hindering clear perception. Another possibility is that while the counselee is nodding and agreeing, and the counselor is nodding and agreeing, each thinks he is in consensus with the other; however, as pointed out in Chapter 2, meanings are in people, not in words. It is possible that each person has interpreted the agreed upon solution differently. For those reasons, closure of the counseling session needs to include a final paraphrase by the counselee that includes action plans. As a result of the session, the counselee should have plans to do something to correct the problem, and both he and the counselor need to be in agreement on what that action is to be.

For nondirective counseling of an employee who has sought out his manager to assist in solving a problem, a written summary including action plans is often useful. Counseling subordinates is a primary responsibility of managers and supervisors, and when they do it well, their subordinates feel closer to them, receive reinforcement, and tend to want to repeat the positive experience. Although counseling subordinates is an important part of the administrative dietitian's job description, there are other things to be done as well. There must be some way for staff to distinguish between which matters are severe enough to take up the manager's time in non-directive counseling and which matters a staff member can settle and solve himself. Insisting that subordinates write up a summary of the session and include specific action plans in a subsequent report not only assures that both have agreed on the solution and action plans, but also gives the employee enough additional work to cause him to think twice before scheduling an appointment for counseling.

Applications of Directive Counseling

Directive counseling is usually not appropriate when working with clients. It is the method used for discussing job-related problems with subordinates when the employee is unaware of the problem, has already been warned about the problem and has not corrected it, or is aware of the problem but hopes that the manager is not. Often, managers tolerate abusive and inappropriate behavior from subordinates, rather than confronting and counseling them directly to improve. Among the reasons for this are the following: the manager may be afraid of handling the counseling poorly and making matters worse; he may be afraid of losing an otherwise good employee if the employee objects to being called in for counseling; he may be afraid of being confronted in return and becoming defensive himself; he may be afraid of retaliation from the employee, either by his spreading stories to the other staff members or by his engaging in some kind of subversive activity on the job; or he may be worried about losing the friendship and respect of the employee. Because directive counseling has the potential to make matters worse, these fears are legitimate for managers who have not had training in directive counseling or in conflict resolution.

Training in directive counseling is essential for managers. Often, individuals who are extraordinary in their professional expertise or ability to perform a professional task are selected to manage others. Promoting a professional expert into management without first providing him with adequate training for the job is like sending an individual to bat with two strikes against him. Directive counseling, like nondirective counseling, can bring two people closer interpersonally, but only when the counselor understands the underlying principles and is sensitive to the need to preserve the self-concept of the counselee.

Managers who fear confronting employees directly and who tolerate poor work behavior may be creating additional morale problems among the rest of the staff. Resentment swells in those who are cooperating and attending to their occupational obligations.

When they see others of equal rank and salary doing less or doing poorly and getting away with it, their own morale sags.

Directive counseling of employees is a form of discipline, and those administering it need to understand the concept. The root of the word "discipline" comes from Latin and means "to train" or "to mold." The attitude of the counselor needs to be that of a caring teacher who wishes to assist the other in improving. As pointed out earlier, the counselee is far more likely to become hostile and defensive in directive counseling than in nondirective counseling, because in directive counseling, he is "called in" rather than doing the "calling," and he may be more concerned with exonerating himself of blame than with collaborating to solve the problem.

Employee Counseling. Employee counseling can be defined as the discussion of a work-related problem to eliminate or reduce it. Problems might include such things as performance and discipline on the job as well as the need for professional and/or skill development. Unless the dietitian has an advanced degree with appropriate clinical counseling experience, counseling his staff should be limited to the occupational concerns mentioned previously and should not include probing into personal problems such as depression, drug abuse, alcoholism, and midlife crisis. For such personal problems, the dietitian should provide referrals, recommending professional therapists, psychologists, or psychiatrists. When employee counseling loses its problem-performance orientation, it runs the risk of being interpreted as meddling or an invasion of privacy.

The administrative dietitian has an obligation to conduct work-related counseling sessions with employees. These should be held as often as necessary, assisting the staff in their professional development as well as dealing with career problems as they occur. Above all, the administrative dietitian should not postpone employee counseling until the annual or semi-annual performance appraisal interviews. Allowing problems to accumulate and handling them all at one time may seem more time-efficient, but in the long run this strategy may be ineffective, for problems may accumulate beyond easy resolutions. Dealing with issues one at a time as they occur is highly advisable.

Guidelines for Directive Counseling. In opening the discussion with the counselee, the counselor must be explicit in his desire to solve a problem rather than to punish. His aim is to improve the subordinate, not to get an apology. One way of keeping the conversation from becoming threatening is to keep remarks performance-centered rather than to make judgments about the staff member. It is more supportive and factual to say, "You have been late six times in the past two weeks," for example, than to say, "Lately you don't seem to care about your job; your attitude is poor." Inferences are not facts. The manager could not possibly know the quality of the employee's "caring" for his job or the condition of his "attitude," but he does know the objective facts—that the employee has been late six times in 2 weeks.

Throughout the interview, the counselor focuses on objective facts, being specific about what he has seen, what he wants in terms of improved behavior, and what action he will take if he does not get it. If others have been complaining, and if the administrative dietitian is unable to document the examples from personal observation, it would be best to postpone the session until he has personal examples. Saying such things as "Some of the staff members have been complaining about your behavior" or "Word has gotten to me" will make the employee suspicious of co-workers and hinder the possibilities for future trusting relationships among the staff.

As in nondirective counseling, the counselor should provide adequate opportunity for the employee to tell his side of the story, and his remarks should be paraphrased as well. As pointed out in the "Count the 'F's' " exercise in Chapter 2, not only do people not know what they do not know, but they easily fall into traps of seeing, hearing, and selectively perceiving what they expect to see and hear. Giving the employee an opportunity to tell his side of the story and then paraphrasing it, and empathizing with what the employee is feeling, usually leads to collaboration in the conflict-resolution process. There may be extenuating circumstances that no one on the staff is aware of that account for the dysfunctional behavior of the employee. Having the employee explain the problem from his perspective may add significant insight and understanding.

When attempts at collaboration do not work, the administrative dietitian can shift to another mode of solving the problem. He can use a win/lose mode, insisting that it be his way "or else." He may win the battle but lose the war if he uses this mode too often. He can back down when he sees the employee becoming defensive and allow the employee to continue the poor performance. He can attempt to compromise with the employee and agree to some exceptions if the employee agrees to improve soon. Too often, however, managers rush to compromise and negotiate behavior change with employees because this approach is less stressful than collaboration. The problem with compromise is that neither party leaves fully satisfied. The employee resents being called on a problem and being asked to change, and the manager resents that he has been unable to bring about the optimal behavior he had originally hoped for. In "real life," there may be times when the best approach is any one of the four discussed previously. Collaboration is not always possible, and so it may be necessary on occasion to use one of the others. Managers, however, need to understand that their first approach should be to try to collaborate on solutions with employees as a first and preferred mode of problem solving.

After an agreement on a solution has been reached, the counselor should describe as specifically as possible what the consequences will be if the agreed upon changes in the employee's behavior are not actualized. At the moment, less tension and a shorter discussion might result from simply saying, "You had better straighten up or else"; however, in the long run, it is far more effective to be exact. One might say, for example, "If you are absent without notice again, I am going to file a warning notice with personnel." The administrative dietitian needs to remember at this point not to exaggerate the consequences or to mention consequences he has not the authority or intention to carry out. If the employee does continue the dysfunctional behavior and the administrative dietitian fails to implement the consequences, the dietitian is implicitly fostering a norm that the others will expect to be applied to them. He is giving one extra chance beyond the final warning. Also, he risks developing the reputation of being "all bark and no bite," and of being an ineffective manager.

If the administrative dietitian has been too lenient in the past, tolerating poor work behavior from the staff and avoiding confrontation in the form of directive counseling, he will encounter resistance if he suddenly insists that everyone must perform optimally. The staff members tend to assume that the supervisor is partially to blame because he did not object to their behavior in the past. In such cases, the counselor needs to admit his share of the blame for his lax supervision in the past. He needs to acknowledge his own responsibility for not attending to the problem sooner, and then to work with the staff on ways of correcting the poor performance.

While verifying understanding is important in nondirective counseling, it is even more important in directive counseling. The tendency for employees to experience physiological stress symptoms from the threat of being called in by the manager heightens the possibility of their misunderstanding some of the communication. Both the administrative dietitian and the staff members need to paraphrase one another to verify that each has understood the other and that they agree on the final solution.

A final step that is appropriate for directive counseling of subordinates is for the administrative dietitian to assure the subordinate that he really does want him to succeed. An expression of confidence and support can help ensure successful implementation of an action plan that both parties have agreed upon. Rather than saying, "Well, let's see what will happen," the dietitian provides more motivation by saying, "I think these are the kinds of ideas that can make a difference." The employee should be reminded that he is an important part of the unit, that the manager does indeed care for him personally, and that his contributions to the staff are valued. If the action plan includes a multi-step process for improvement, it would be wise to set follow-up dates for meeting with the subordinate. Doing so not only confirms commitment, but also adds incentive to begin changes.

The processes of both directive and nondirective counseling are far more effective if a trusting relationship exists between the counselor and counselee. In the case of directive counseling between a manager and a subordinate, there is an ongoing and consistent relationship before the counseling as well as after it. The manager cannot vacillate between being unfeeling, bureaucratic, officious, and cold toward subordinates most of the time and being suddenly supportive, caring, and trustworthy during the counseling session. Subordinates begin inferring the degree of trustworthiness and caring on the part of the manager from the time of their first encounter with him, with each subsequent encounter adding to their perceptions. Being a manager of other people is actually a "helping profession" in itself. The manager needs to lay the foundation for that trust early and continuously. Directive counseling is characterized by being both a caring and a determined effort to correct dysfunctional behavior affecting work performance.

As in nondirective counseling, the manager must attend to the supporting nonverbal behavior throughout the directive counseling interview. He should select a private place free of interruptions. The spatial dynamics of the location should allow the two people to feel close and intimate as feelings are being shared and help is being given to solve the problem. The manager needs to act, talk, look, and gesture in a manner that allows the subordinate to infer that the purpose of the counseling session is to change dysfunctional behavior, not to reject or punish him. Finally, the manager has to remember to allow adequate time for full expression of thoughts, scheduling multiple sessions when appropriate.

COMPONENTS OF NUTRITIONAL COUNSELING

The overall process of nutritional counseling is generally divided into three separate functions: interviewing, counseling, and consulting. Interviewing, discussed in Chapter 3, involves the gathering of information and requires considerable training to elicit accurately the selective information vital to the counseling process. Counseling, per se, is a process involving listening, accepting, clarifying, and helping the client to form his own conclusions and develop his own plan of action. The dietitian guides the client's thinking to focus on objectives, interprets and evaluates information, and translates for the patient the regimen prescribed by the physician. In addition to adding to and enhancing the knowledge and understanding of the client, consulting involves developing plans or proposals for a client, based on observations and evaluations.

Nutritional counseling is a process that assists an individual in learning about himself, about his eating habits as part of his total environment, and about methods of coping with his dietary problems. The purpose of counseling is to change behavior, which requires both learning and motivation. In the person with diabetes, for example, the purpose of nutritional counseling would be to change from current to diabetic eating patterns. For the pregnant woman, the purpose might be to add to the diet foods that meet the nutrient needs of pregnancy while maintaining appropriate caloric levels. Nutritional counseling involves deliberation and collaboration between two parties (the dietitian or counselor and the client or counselee) during which values may be examined, knowledge imparted and acquired, new ways of dealing with life situations learned, goals set, and decisions made. The counselee is assisted in setting goals and in planning new and different actions.

Since the purpose of counseling is to promote change, or to select and implement new food-related behaviors, the dietitian should note that change is never easy for people. Continuing with one's current, comfortable lifestyle and avoiding change represent the path of least resistance. Resistance to change may occur at an unrecognized, subconscious level and should be expected and probed by the counselor. Changing one's eating patterns is probably one of the most difficult lifestyle changes an individual has to make, owing to the fact that dietary habits are long standing, have been associated with pleasure from the time mother offered the bottle or the breast, and may provide psychological relief for emotions such as boredom, frustration, and stress. At the same time, food may be associated with status, comfort, security, and celebration.

A number of models of the nutritional counseling process may be found in the literature.[11-18] Models help one to examine and understand the steps in a complex process. The following model is a composite of those available. For further examination of nutritional counseling, which is beyond the scope of this book, other sources are recommended.[14,17,19] The components of nutritional counseling include the following:

1. Preparation
2. Assessment: dietary, behavioral, physical, social, and cognitive environments
3. Treatment
4. Evaluation
5. Follow-up

Preparation. The first step is to gather in advance data or information about the client that may have an impact on treatment and to arrange the physical environment for effective counseling. The physical environment was discussed earlier in the text.

In a hospital or clinical setting, the medical record is the source of data about the patient. Height, weight, results of laboratory tests, and medical problems should be noted. Mason suggests a number of factors that may affect eating patterns, including family status, occupation, income, educational level, ethnicity, religion, physical activity and recreation, physical disabilities or impairments, and place of residence.[15] Information that is unavailable from the medical record may be obtained during the interview. The diet counselor is expected to know the client physiologically, psychologically, socially, and economically, i.e., he should know what factors make the client what he is.[11] The counselor must view the client as an individual living and interacting in an environment that influences his motivation and capabilities.

A second source of data is one's own records kept from previous counseling sessions or previous contact with the client. These records should be reviewed prior to follow-up counseling.

Assessment. Since the purpose of counseling is to promote change, the dietitian needs to collect and assess data that indicate what changes need to be made and what personal and lifestyle factors may promote or interfere with changes in eating patterns. After informing the client of the purpose of the interview ("I need to collect some information in order to understand your problem and assist you with it"), and after establishing good rapport with the client, the dietitian may collect data from the client by using the interviewing skills discussed in Chapter 3.

The assessment may have a number of important functions. These include making both parties aware of dietary habits and health history, providing baseline information from which to gauge process, alerting both parties to the demands placed on the patient so that realistic goals can be set, providing both parties with ideas for making changes, providing an opportunity to continue rapport, and enabling the counselor and client to work together on a plan for gradual changes that are congruent with the client's lifestyle.[17]

The dietitian may collect data on current eating habits as described in Chapter 3, and on the physicial, social, and cognitive environments.[19] Behavioral assessment is discussed in Chapter 5. The physical environment includes where meals are eaten (at home or in restaurants and in which rooms of the home) and events that occur while eating (watching television). The social environment, which may or may not be supportive, includes family, friends, social norms and trends involved with eating behaviors (e.g., popular food customs of a bridge club, drinking buddies).

The cognitive or mental environment involves the client's thoughts and feelings about food, self-image, and confidence. It concerns what the client says to himself about his food intake and life since personal thoughts may or may not promote successful change. Some thoughts may be positive, such as "I love a steak and baked potato," or "My favorite snacks are potato chips and beer." There may be negative and self-defeating thoughts, or thoughts of failure, boredom, stress, or hunger. Examples include "It's too difficult"; "It's not worth it"; "I can't do it"; "I've been on diets before, always failed, and regained all of the weight I lost"; or "I'm happy the way I am and don't want to change." Since behavior is influenced by beliefs and attitudes, one may need to explore these in relation to medical condition, nutrition, diets, and health.

After the data are gathered, they should be analyzed and interpreted. Influences on eating patterns should be identified, and recommended changes noted. Changes may be thought of as problems to be solved with the client. This information is considered baseline data of the client prior to counseling and should be recorded later and referred to in future counseling sessions.

Treatment. Treatment involves a number of substeps, which include the following:

1. Explaining the counseling relationship.
2. Identifying the problems—The difference between what is eaten and what should be eaten determines what the client needs to do and where change is needed.
3. Exploring the problems, conditions, circumstances, and setting of priorities for change with the client.
4. Setting goals for change with the client and eliciting a commitment.

The counseling relationship has been described previously in the chapter. The counselor may wish to clarify that the responsibility for change rests with the client, but that he is willing to be of assistance in solving problems and making new plans.

Before problems are explored, it is probably advisable to discuss with the client, and show approval for, those current food choices that do not need changing, i.e., what he is already doing right according to the diet prescription. Problems—foods that should be omitted, or food or cooking practices that should be changed—may be discussed next, perhaps starting with the dietitian's estimation of what is most important. The conditions and circumstances surrounding food behaviors need to be explored. This stage of counseling requires the skills of the helping-process model discussed earlier: listening, questioning, accepting, clarifying, and helping the client find solutions to his problems and develop his own plan of action.[11] Counseling should not be directed solely at the client's knowledge, but also at feelings, attitudes, beliefs, and values, which have strong and powerful influences on dietary behaviors. Knowledge is a tool only if and when an individual is ready to change.[20]

At the resolving stage, one or two priorities for change should be selected for the next week or so. Clients who are enthusiastic about making total changes immediately are setting themselves up for frustration and possible failure, which may lead to abandoning the dietary changes altogether. The counselor should guard against this. Slow, steady changes that will persist over time are preferable. It is important to discuss the problems thoroughly, along with the impact of physical, social, and cognitive environments on the problems selected for change. Because the client is the one who has to make the changes, he is the one who must decide what changes to make. Having the client select the particular changes increases his motivation and commitment. The counselor may wish to guide the individual toward those goals that seem easier to accomplish. The goal is for the client to have a successful change experience before returning for follow-up counseling. Success with first assignments is especially important when the cognitive environment is negative. "What one or two changes can you try this week?" "What are your thoughts about making those changes?" "What things might interfere with doing it?" The dietitian can ask questions to help the client decide what to do.

To set goals for change, ask the client to explain what he intends to do during the next week and why he believes it is important. Ask if there are problems in doing it, and if there are, discuss them. Tell the client to expect some problems since some things will not have been considered. If he is aware of the possibility of problems beforehand, the client may avoid abandoning the diet with the first sign of difficulty. Supplying him with your phone number for asking questions may also resolve this problem.

The dietitian may wish to know if there are others with whom the client can discuss the goals since a public commitment may make it more likely for goals to be accomplished.[19] The dietitian may ask the client to keep records of food intake and environments, which he should bring to the next appointment as a way for him and the counselor to learn about factors affecting eating behavior, and as a demonstration of his commitment to change.[13] The client's personal records, observations, and analysis of his environment contribute to his understanding. Chapter 5, "Behavior Modification," discusses this matter in more detail. By the end of the counseling session, the client should not only know what to do and how to do it, but also want to do it.[21] The client has to perceive and accept the need for change. Motivation for change should be explored, and present dangers in continuing his current dietary patterns should be anticipated and discussed. The counseling process involves more than distributing printed diet materials to clients.

Evaluation. The dietitian may wish to evaluate both the success of the client in following new dietary behaviors and his own personal skills as a counselor. Counselor self-evaluation forms may be found in the literature.[17] Rethinking the session may be helpful. Records of the problems and goals, and of the factors influencing them, should be kept by the dietitian for future measurement of client change, and documentation of the counseling is completed on the medical record. A measure of success such as weight lost in an obese person is obvious. Changes in laboratory values, such as blood sugar levels in people with diabetes or cholesterol and lipid levels of cardiovascular patients, are more difficult to evaluate, since they depend on factors beyond dietary compliance.

Follow-Up. Frequent follow-up for reassessment and support is essential until the client is self-sufficient. Discussion at subsequent sessions should focus first on what went well, i.e., the successful experiences. Such positive focus helps the client feel that he can have some control over his eating, health, and life. Records kept by the client should be examined jointly and discussed, and problems should be solved. Overlooking the records indicates to the client that they were not considered important. If things are going well, new goals for change may be established jointly. Support and reinforcement to strengthen desirable habits, along with gradual, planned changes, should continue as long as necessary.

Enthusiasm for change may decline the first week and even more the second week, as problems develop. Therefore, frequent follow-up appointments should be scheduled. Dietitians in tertiary care settings who do not have the opportunity for follow-up may need to refer patients to clinical dietitians in outpatient clinics or in private practice, since one session with a client is insufficient to promote long-term change in health counseling. The minimal requirements for a successful nutritional counseling program and long-term change are active patient participation in the planning, execution, and evaluation of various nutritional change strategies, continuity of care over an extended period, and treatment strategies tailored to the individual's needs.[13]

COUNSELING AS A SPECIALIZATION FOR DIETITIANS

The concept of the intervention specialist is emerging as a challenge to dietitians who want to expand their role to include counseling patients on therapeutic regimens in matters other than diet. Articles have begun to appear in the dietetic literature suggesting that the dietitian can prepare to counsel clients in other areas. The concept originated in clinical trials, where dietitians effectively counseled study participants on adherence to taking drugs as well as on adherence to diet. Counseling in areas of stress management, exercise, and smoking cessation are other examples. Requirements of education and experience for intervention specialists are essentially the same as those for registered dietitians; the only difference is that additional training in interviewing and behavior counseling may be needed.[12] Intervention specialists do require, of course, more time with the patient than the usual one or two counseling sessions afforded to clinical dietitians. The dietitian needs extra time in this counseling approach to achieve long-term healthy behavior in cases of adherence problems.

Dietitians need to train for this role and to promote it as being of significant benefit to private physicians and their patients. One writer urges dietitians to educate the medical community about their qualifications as intervention specialists and their entitlement to increased professional responsibility.[12] The intervention specialist can also coordinate several different prescribed treatments that require behavior changes by the patient. Currently, drug, diet, smoking cessation, and physical therapy treatments are often prescribed with no provision for monitoring success of their incorporation into a client's lifestyle. Close cooperation and coordination between the patient, the intervention specialist, and other members of the medical team can help improve the quality of medical care.[22]

All dietitians need to be knowledgeable in the concepts, processes, and techniques of counseling although they may apply them in different situations in professional practice. Some clinical dietitians, with added training, are expanding their roles to those of intervention specialists dealing with long-term health behavior problems in addition to diet, and they are counseling to achieve patient adherence. Chapter 5 discusses another approach to counseling, that of behavior modification.

SUGGESTED ACTIVITIES

1. During the next week, make arrangements to view a dietitian's counseling session, noting particularly what occurs during stage I, *involving*. What behavior on the part of the dietitian facilitates the building of rapport and trust?

2. During the following week, make three efforts to express caring for another using nonverbal behavior. What do you do, and how does the other respond?

3. Using a videotape recorder, meet with another individual and record 10 minutes of interaction and conversation. Comment on the quality of your verbal and nonverbal behavior. What kind of messages might one infer from your demeanor?

4. In groups of three, develop a conversation around the topics presented in this chapter. Before one person can respond to what

another has said, however, he will need to paraphrase to the other's satisfaction what the other has just said.

5. During the next week, practice paraphrasing after others talk. What reactions do you get? Does your paraphrasing tend to cause the other to go on talking?

6. In round-robin groups of 5, each person expresses a statement, and the person to the right should attempt to identify a feeling expressed in the statement. After three rounds, discuss the reactions of the group to the attempts at empathizing.

7. Write both a paraphrase and empathic comment to the following comments made by a counselee:
    A. I feel awkward discussing my eating habits. I feel I must be disgusting to you.
    B. People tend to think I'm jolly, but I don't believe they take me seriously.
    C. I am at a point now where I don't believe I will ever lose the weight.

8. Form triads consisting of a counselor, counselee, and observer. Each individual should take a turn in each of the roles for 7 minutes. The counselee should play the role of an obese client, and the counselor should use paraphrasing and empathizing, along with open and closed questions, to facilitate disclosure and problem solving. After each round, the observer should share his reactions to the counselor's approach and encourage feedback from the counselee to the counselor. From the counselee's perspective, what did the counselor do that helped their interaction; what did he do that hindered it?

9. Write an open-ended question for each of the statements below:
    A. I never have any fun at family gatherings anymore. Being on this diet has taken the fun out of my life.
    B. I dislike my supervisor at work. No matter what I do, he criticizes me.
    C. Since I developed these health problems, it seems that all I do is think about my diet.

10. Meet with someone who is not in the class and discuss with him your motivations for wanting to counsel clients. Which of your personal needs might be satisfied in helping others?

11. After each of the statements below, write responses in the form of a closed-ended question, an open-ended question, or a directive.

A. My work situation is impossible. It seems that I'm the scapegoat for everybody. I'm beginning to wonder if I should consider looking for another job.

B. It doesn't seem fair to me that I should have to work weekends when the staff members who have been here only two years longer don't have to.

C. It seems easy every morning to promise myself that today I will stick to the program you designed for me. By noon, however, I begin thinking that I'll never be able to comply with the diet for the rest of my life, so why bother?

REFERENCES

1. A New Look at the Profession of Dietetics. Chicago, American Dietetic Assoc. 1985.
2. Baird, S., and Armstrong, R.: Role Delineation for Entry Level Clinical Dietetics. Chicago, American Dietetic Assoc., 1981.
3. Baird, S., and Sylvester, J.: Role Delineation and Verification for Entry-Level Positions in Community Dietetics. Chicago, American Dietetic Assoc. 1983.
4. Baird, S., and Sylvester, J: Role Delineation and Verification for Entry-Level Positions in Foodservice Systems Management. Chicago, American Dietetic Assoc. 1983.
5. Rogers, C.: Client-Centered Therapy. Boston, Houghton Mifflin, 1951.
6. Rogers, C.: On Becoming a Person. Boston, Houghton Mifflin, 1961.
7. Patterson, C.H. Theories of Counseling and Psychotherapy. New York, Harper & Row, 1966.
8. Rogers, C.: The interpersonal relationship: The core of guidance. Harvard Educational Review, *32*:416, 1962.
9. Danish, S., D'Augelli, A., and Hauer, A.: Helping Skills: A Basic Training Program. Trainee's Workbook. 2nd ed. New York, Human Sciences Press, 1980.
10. Kinlaw, D.: Helping Skills for Human Resource Development: A Facilitator's Package. San Diego, University Associates, 1981.
11. Ling, L., Spragg, D., Stein, P., and Myers, M.: Guidelines for diet counseling. J. Am. Diet. Assoc., *6*:571, 1975.
12. Pace, P., Russell, M., Probstfield, J., and Insull, W.: Intervention specialist: New role for dietitians' counseling skills. J. Am. Diet. Assoc., *84*:1357, 1984.
13. Zifferblatt, S., and Wilbur, C.: Dietary counseling: Some realistic expectations and guidelines. J. Am. Diet. Assoc., *70*:591, 1977.
14. Snetselaar, L.: Nutrition Counseling Skills: Assessment, Treatment, and Evaluation. Rockville, MD, Aspen Publications, 1983.
15. Mason, M., Wenberg, B., and Welsch, P.: The Dynamics of Clinical Dietetics. 2nd. ed. New York, John Wiley and Sons, 1982.
16. Schrott, H., and Snetselaar, L.: Building Nutrition Counseling Skills, Vol II. Washington, DC, U.S. Dept. of Health and Human Services, 1984.
17. Rabb, C., and Tillotson, J. (eds): Heart to Heart. Washington, DC, U.S. Dept. of Health and Human Services, 1983.
18. Wiley, J.: Growth process in nutrition counseling. J. Am. Diet. Assoc., *69*:505, 1976.
19. Wilbur, C.: Nutrition Counseling Skills, ACS 5. Chicago, American Dietetic Assoc., 1980.
20. Hay, A.: Factors influencing the counseling behavior of clinical dietitians. Doctoral dissertation. University of Tennessee, Knoxville, 1983.
21. Mahoney, M., and Caggiula, A.: Applying behavioral methods to nutritional counseling. J. Am. Diet. Assoc., *72*:372, 1978.
22. Franz, M.: The dietitian: A key member of the diabetes team. J. Am. Diet. Assoc., *84*:285, 1984.

5 _____ Ann B. Williams, Ph.D.

Behavior Modification

There is one characteristic that is common to all living organisms—behavior. The behavior of some organisms is simple, limited, and to many of us, quite unexciting. The behavior of other organisms, such as human beings, is complex, sophisticated, extensive, and to most people, quite exciting and interesting, however difficult it may be to understand. One of the first questions that a scientist asks to understand an organism is, "What does it do?"

When it has been determined what an organism does, that is, how it behaves, the behaviors are categorized as being primarily innate (inherited), or primarily learned (acquired). The more interesting and complex behaviors of human beings are learned behaviors, although certainly even complex learned behaviors are subject to the limitations of one's genetic endowment.

According to Stunkard, "People are best described by their behavior—what they think, feel, and do in specific situations."[1] Since they are learned or acquired, many human behaviors can be changed or modified. One of the tasks of the discipline of psychology has been to attempt to establish the principles that underlie the process of behavioral change or modification.

For years, the approach of psychologists to this task has been largely based on environment. Behaviors are thought to be acquired or learned through interaction with the environment. Because of this strong environmental orientation, much attention has been devoted to the study of the basic principles of learning. The position taken is that if many behaviors can be, and indeed, are learned, then these same behaviors could also be "unlearned." There is then tremendous potential for behavioral change.

This chapter reviews the principles of learning and behavior modification that have evolved from research studies. Included are classical conditioning, operant or instrumental conditioning based on positive reinforcement or rewards, and observational learning or modelng after others' behavior. The role of cognitions, the individual's mental perceptions of events, and their effect on behavior, a newer area of research, is included.

In behavior modification, the therapist attempts to alter previously learned behavior or to encourage the development of new behavior.

Food and eating behaviors are deeply seated in the individual and may be resistant to change. Furnishing information concerning what to eat frequently is insufficient in promoting alterations in eating behaviors or adherence to modified diets. In addition to information on nutrition, behavior modification principles may be used, as they offer the dietitian another approach to counseling.

Applications of behavior modification principles as part of the treatment of various nutritional problems are examined in this chapter. One of the earliest and the most frequently used applications was to the treatment of obesity. Therapy for eating disorders such as anorexia nervosa, bulimia, diabetes mellitus, and cardiovascular diseases are other potential uses of behavior modification.

In personnel management, supervisors may be interested in altering the behavior of subordinates and encouraging the develoment of new behaviors. Although the term behavior modification as applied to employees may sound manipulative, the principles may be used by an honest and understanding supervisor who has told employees what he is doing. These principles are the basis for the advice in the book *The One Minute Manager*.[2] Modeling has been used in employee training programs.

CLASSICAL CONDITIONING

The methods of behavior modification are based on principles of learning that, for the most part, have been discovered in the experimental laboratory. According to Hill, the best known animals in the history of psychology were the dogs housed in the laboratory of Ivan Pavlov, the Russian physiologist, who was conducting research on digestive processes.[3] Serendipitously, Pavlov noted that his laboratory animals salivated not only when food was presented, but also when the laboratory assistant, who regularly fed them, came into the room; at times, they even salivated at the sound of the laboratory door opening. Pavlov spent the rest of his life investigating a type of learning based on association, now known as classical conditioning.

Pavlov realized immediately that the response of salivation to laboratory assistants and noisy doors was not a part of the physiological make-up of the dog. The dogs were salivating when events occurred that had regularly and repeatedly come before the presentation of their food. An association was apparently being formed between some event and the future appearance of food.

Pavlov noted that certain environmental events or stimuli would reliably trigger or elicit a particular behavioral response. For example, food in a dog's mouth would reliably produce saliva. The triggering event (food in the mouth) became known as the unconditioned stimulus (US), while the response that was triggered (salivation) was called the unconditioned response (UR). This relationship was built into the organism, and hence, was unconditioned. Conditioning occurs, then, when some other stimulus (a neutral stimulus) that originally does not trigger the particular response (salivation) eventually comes to produce that response. This occurs by pairing the originally neutral stimulus with the unconditioned stimulus. When conditioning has occurred, the conditioned stimulus (CS), which was originally neutral, produces a response that is the same as, or very similar to, the US. In the example, the CS was the presence of the laboratory assistant. Pavlov showed that bells, tones, lights, and many other stimuli could serve as the CS and could come to elicit the response of salivation, which is labeled a conditioned response (CR) once it is triggered by or produced by a CS.

Many different types of responses have been found to be responsive to classical conditioning principles. Not only reflexive responses, such as salivation and eye blinking, but also complex emotional responses can be classically conditioned, as illustrated by the following example. The heart pounds, and beads of perspiration appear on the forehead as one hears the siren of an ambulance approaching a neighbor's home. The same phenomenon may occur when the teacher passes out examination questions. Try to construct a scenario to account for this response in terms of classical conditioning principles, or think of other situations where classical conditioning might play a part in human behavior or emotional responses.

OPERANT CONDITIONING

At about the same time that Pavlov was delineating the principles of classical conditioning, a young American scientist, Edward Thorndike, was pursuing the investigation of learning principles from another perspective. Thorndike used many types of animals and designed and constructed "puzzle boxes" for cats. A hungry cat was placed inside the box with food located outside. To have access to the food, the cat had to solve the puzzle of how to escape from the box. Thorndike observed that the cats made trial-and-error responses until escape was achieved and the food consumed. Gradually, the time required to solve the puzzle decreased, and the behavior that achieved success in solving the puzzle became dominant, while nonsuccessful behaviors were eliminated.

Thorndike proposed an explanation for this phenomenon based on a principle he called the Law of Effect. The Law of Effect stated that behaviors could be changed by their consequences. Responses that were followed by satisfying consequences would be stamped in or strengthened. Behaviors not followed by satisfying consequences, or behaviors followed by annoying consequences, would be weakened and less likely to occur in the future. Thorndike's Law of Effect led to much research in principles of learning and formed the foundation for the study of operant or instrumental conditioning, which is learning or conditioning based on reinforcement or reward.

The focal point of research on the Law of Effect is the relationship between responses, or behaviors, and the consequences of those behaviors. Schwartz described four types of response-consequence outcomes.[4] First, responses or behaviors may produce positive outcomes, a consequence known as positive reinforcement. An example would be the lavish praise and attention one receives after achieving a svelte new figure. Second, responses may produce negative outcomes; this consequence is known as punishment. Punishment decreases the future likelihood of a response. Examples of punishment include the receipt of a traffic ticket for an improper left turn and the inability to fit into a favorite, expensive outfit after gaining weight. Third, responses may result in the elimination or removal of aversive stimuli that are already present. This consequence is known as negative reinforcement or escape, and it is similar to positive reinforcement in that it increases the future likelihood or probability of a response. Examples include escaping devastating cold by going into a heated building, escaping a poor television show by changing channels, and escaping unfavorable comparisons with others by shaping and trimming one's figure. Finally, responses may prevent an aversive event from occurring. Examples include avoiding the cold by staying indoors and avoiding unfavorable comparisons with others by maintaining a trim figure. The avoidance of aversive events increases the future likelihood of the response, as does positive reinforcement. Behaviors that are not positively reinforced or negatively reinforced, leading to escape or avoidance of aversive stimuli, should not increase in strength, and with continued nonreinforcement, should decrease in strength.

Later behaviorists continued where Thorndike concluded. B.F. Skinner is best known for his championing of a set of methods and terms to explain behavior on the basis of the principles of operant conditioning. Skinner developed a situation in which behavior could be observed in discrete units and subsequently recorded. This situation was an operant chamber, which has been dubbed a "Skinner box." The lever presses of rats and key pecks of pigeons have been the most frequently studied responses. Skinner's enthusiasm for the behavioristic approach was not limited to lower animals, however, for he proposed wide application for the principles that were established. In recent years, the behavioristic approach has become an increasingly important practical technique in many settings, such as classrooms, mental hospitals, prisons, clinics, the work place, and self-management situations.

MODELING

In addition to classical and operant conditioning as modes of behavior change, a third form of learning is known as observational learning, or modeling. Learning by modeling involves the observation of some behavior or pattern of behaving, which is followed later by the performance of either the same or some similar behavior. Albert Bandura is associated closely with this method of learning by modeling.

The model being observed may be either another person or a representation of the pattern of behaving. The model, then, could be another human, an animal, or some symbolic representation that uses verbal stimuli, such as films, television, or other media presentations.

The effectiveness of learning by modeling appears to be directly related to certain characteristics of the model. The two characteristics found to be most relevant are the observer's similarity to the model and the status of the model. The more similar the characteristics of the model are to those of the observer, the higher is the probability that learning by modeling will occur. Research has shown that models with greater status, prestige, or expertise are more likely to be imitated by the observer than models lacking these characteristics. Tennis players, for example, are more likely to imitate the two-handed backhand technique of Chris Evert-Lloyd than a technique of an unknown player. Certainly, this fact has been noted and capitalized on by all of the movie and television stars and other well-known persons who have produced books and videotapes of their fitness/exercise/nutrition programs. Many people model their behavior after the person with "status" even though equally effective or superior programs could be developed by relatively unknown, but professionally trained, nutritionists and exercise physiologists.

To take advantage of modeling, clinical dietitians may try sharing success stories of people who have made permanent dietary modifications for the benefit of their health. In group therapy, clients who have followed their diets may serve as models for others. The dietitian may be viewed as a model by the client. As a result, in counseling obese people, the counselor should be of normal weight, and dietitians should be following the normal nutrition recommendations that they give to others.

Behavior modeling is used in employee training programs to teach basic supervisory techniques, selling skills, and various other verbal skills through observation of films and videotapes. In assigning a new employee to work with a current employee, the latter serves as a model. Managers should make sure that their own behaviors are exemplary of what they expect of subordinates.[5] If the supervisor adds an extra 10 minutes to the allowed time for a coffee break, for example, employees may model their own behavior after this example.

Today there is no doubt that a great deal of human learning or behavior change is due to modeling, even though traditionally, emphasis has been placed on the stimulus-response (or behavior-consequence) approach to explaining changes in behavior, or on the acquisition and extinction of responses.[3] These three approaches—classical conditioning, operant conditioning, and modeling—form the basis for behavior modification. The behavioristic position is that many behaviors are learned or are alterable through the use of these three learning principles.

COGNITIVE PSYCHOLOGY

In behavior modification, one attempts to alter behaviors that previously have been learned or to encourage the development of new behaviors. More recently, the importance of cognitive psychology has been recognized. Researchers have considered the role of cognitions and have emphasized the role of cognitive and symbolic processes in influencing behaviors. It has been noted that an individual's perceptions of external events, rather than the events themselves, often account for behaviors.[7] The client's thought patterns, beliefs, attitudes, opinions, and thoughts about himself may affect change.

The counselor needs to explore *cognitions,* which may be defined as what the person says to himself. Since many overweight individuals have had previous unsuccessful experiences with dietary control, they may have feelings of low self-worth, personal failure, or guilt, which can interfere with successful dietary change and weight loss. The person may have self-critical thoughts, such as "I'm a pig," "I look so fat," or "I can't lose weight and am a failure." With all clients, the dietitian should look for negative cognitions, such as "This diet is too difficult," "I can't do it," "I don't see why this is important," or "I'd rather eat what I want and die happy." When the dietitian discovers negative cognitions, he should discuss these with the client. Cognitive restructuring is used to modify negative, self-defeating, or pessimistic thoughts into more positive ones that will assist the patient with dietary adherence. The client should be encouraged to "accentuate the positive," congratulate himself for any progress—however small—and counter negative thoughts with constructive ones that will help him to cope.

CHANGING EATING BEHAVIORS

As the principles that govern behavior and behavior change became more clearly defined, it was increasingly apparent that nutritionists and behavioral scientists should work together to provide methods of using these principles in applied settings where changes in dietary habits are the primary goal. The National Heart, Lung, and Blood Institute has been one of the leaders in encouraging this type of collaboration.[8] The most frequent application has been the behavioral management of obesity, but cooperative programs have led to applications in such diverse areas of concern as cardiovascular disease, eating disorders, and diabetes mellitus.

Dietary behaviors must be studied in relation to the client's total environment, which includes physical, social, psychological, and physiological factors, as well to all conditions and events that precede and follow eating. Several behavioral scientists have referred to this framework as the ABCs, derived from analysis of the *antecedents* (stimuli or cues) of behavior, the *behavior* (response) itself, and the *consequences* (reinforcement or reward) of the behavior.[1,9] For example, seeing a package of cookies left on the kitchen counter may be the antecedent or cue. The behavior is eating half a package of cookies in the kitchen when one is home alone at 4:00 P.M. The consequences may be pleasure from the taste of the cookies and reduced feelings of hunger or frustration with increased feelings of happiness and satisfaction, which reinforce the behavior. The dietitian and the client must find ways to decrease undesirable eating behaviors and increase new, desirable ones.

Antecedents. Behavior modification techniques work by regulating the antecedents, the behavior of eating itself, and the consequences or rewards. Analysis of antecedents of behavior seeks to control or limit the stimuli or cues to eating. For example, a cue may be seeing or smelling food, watching television, arriving home from work or school, attending a social event, or noticing the presence of extra food on the table at mealtime. Behavior may be influenced by both internal and external factors. There may be internal cues, such as physiological feelings of hunger or psychological feelings of loneliness or boredom. A number of external variables may cue eating, such as noting the time of day or passing an ice cream shop on the street. Both internal and external factors may be mediated by cognitive factors, such as not caring about current weight levels or not wishing to dull one's appetite for the next meal.[10]

The strategy involves decreasing the number of times the person is exposed to situations where he consumes food. A list of suggestions for changing behavior that have been recommended by various authors for persons desiring to lose weight is found in Figure 5-1.[1,11,12] To modify antecedents, the dietitian may suggest removing negative cues (not buying improper foods), introducing new, more positive cues (exercising instead of eating), restricting behavior to one set of cues (eating only at designated times), cognitive restructuring discussed previously, and role-playing new responses to old antecedents (telling a friend you would rather go to a movie

BEHAVIOR MODIFICATION TECHNIQUES

I. PROVIDE INCENTIVES TO AID PATIENTS IN MAINTAINING COMMITMENT
   A. Determine ways to focus attention on successful experiences. A positive comment by the counselor is helpful, and one can always find something positive to say.
   B. Encourage people to tell others about dietary goals. This public commitment often will aid in maintaining one's course of action.
   C. Have the person anticipate problems that might come up and consider possible solutions before a problem arises. Having a plan ready will make focusing on the goal easier.
   D. Concentrate on allowed foods and portions, rather than the disallowed. Be positive.
   E. Keep reminding the person that dietary change is a gradual process. Dietary habits were not developed in a brief period of time and probably will not be significantly changed in a short time. Set realistic goals for immediate and long-term change. Encourage successive approximations to the desired behavior.

II. LEARN EATING HABITS (AND EXERCISE HABITS) BY RECORD KEEPING
   One cannot change a habit until one knows what it is. Self-monitoring with accurate records of the foods consumed is necessary for behavioral control of eating. Information to consider recording would be:
   A. What food was eaten
   B. Quantity of each food
   C. What the person was doing just prior to eating (to help identify cues)
   D. Place of eating (cue providing)
   E. With whom eating occurs, or alone (cue providing)
   F. How the person felt (cue providing)
   G. Time of eating (cue providing)
This record keeping exercise can identify the person's patterns of food intake and those cues that are associated with food consumption as well as the emotional outcome of eating. The person will become more aware of the environmental stimuli that are associated with eating behavior.

III. CONTROL THE STIMULI (CUES) AND RESTRUCTURE THE ENVIRONMENT
   A. Physical environment:
      1. Based on the records kept, have the person identify physical stimuli in the environment that are associated with, and therefore are cues to, inappropriate eating behaviors. Different stimuli become associated with the act of eating and can become signals for appropriate or inappropriate food consumption.
      2. Ask the person to identify physical stimuli that could remind him to eat properly. Examples of these would be charts or graphs, cartoons, signs, and the like. The presence of appropriate foods in the home will probably be the best cue to appropriate eating, supplemented by the elimination of inappropriate foods.

Fig. 5-1. Techniques for behavior modification. (Adapted from Stunkard, A., and Berthold, H.: What is behavior therapy? Am. J. Clin. Nutr., 41:821, 1985; Rabb, C., and Tillotson, J.L. (eds.): Heart to Heart. Washington, DC, U.S. Dept. of Health and Human Services, 1983; and Fensterheim, H., and Baer, J.: Don't Say Yes When You Want to Say No. New York, Dell Pub. Co., 1975.)

3. Have the person specify a special place where food should be consumed, such as at the dining table, and not in front of the television set or kitchen sink.
4. Make those foods that are acceptable in the nutrition plan as attractive as possible. Use good dishes, crystal, and so forth to make dining a pleasant event.
5. Set up shopping trips based on the following suggestions:
    a. shop for food only after eating
    b. use a shopping list
    c. avoid ready-to-eat foods
    d. do not carry more money than needed for shopping list
6. Set up specific plans and activities
    a. substitute exercise for snacking
    b. eat meals and snacks at scheduled times
    c. do not accept food offered by others
    d. store food out of sight
    e. remove food from inappropriate storage areas in the house
    f. use smaller dishes
    g. avoid being the food server
    h. leave the table immediately after eating
    i. discard leftovers
7. Regarding special events and holidays
    a. drink fewer alcoholic beverages
    b. plan eating before parties
    c. eat a low calorie snack before parties
    d. practice polite ways to decline food
    e. do not get discouraged by occasional setbacks

B. Social environment
   1. Have the person identify the types of social situations which contribute to poor eating habits. Examples of stimuli in the social environment that might contribute to difficulty for the person would be negative statements from family members or friends, social situations where there are expectations for eating inappropriate or disallowed foods.
   2. Have the person identify the kind of social interactions that would be supportive of good eating habits and following the nutrition plan. Role playing can be useful with the person practicing how he will ask others to help him change his eating habits.

C. Cognitive or mental environment
   1. Have the person identify what thoughts and feelings are likely to make attempts to change eating habits unsuccessful.
   2. After the person has identified possible negative thoughts that could lead to discouragement, help him develop some positive thoughts that can be used to counteract the negative ones.
   3. Avoid setting unreasonable goals.

IV. CHANGE ACTUAL EATING BEHAVIOR
   A. Slow down
      1. Take one small bite at a time
      2. Put the fork down between mouthfuls
      3. Chew thoroughly before swallowing
      4. Take a break during the meal. Stop eating completely for a short period.
   B. Leave some food on the plate

Fig. 5-1. (Continued)

C. Make eating of inappropriate foods as difficult as possible
D. Control snacks
   1. Save allowable foods from meals for snacks
   2. Establish behaviors incompatible with eating
   3. Prepare snacks the way one prepares meals—on a plate
   4. Keep a quantity of low calorie foods, such as raw vegetables, on hand to use. Have them ready to eat and easy to get.
E. Instruct the person that when he eats, he should not be performing any other act. The cues associated with eating should be restricted to that act, so one should not eat while reading, sewing, watching television, and so on.
F. Have the person continue monitoring himself

V. CHANGE EXERCISE BEHAVIOR
   A. Routine activity
      1. Increase routine activity
      2. Increase use of stairs
      3. Keep records of distance walked daily
   B. Exercise
      1. Begin supervised exercise program under specialist's direction
      2. Keep records of daily exercise
      3. Increase exercise gradually

VI. SET UP A REWARD AND REINFORCEMENT SYSTEM
   A. Have family and friends provide this help in the form of praise and material rewards.
   B. Clearly define behaviors to be reinforced
   C. Use self-monitoring records as a basis for rewards
   D. Plan specific rewards for specific behaviors. Use written contracts.
   E. Gradually make rewards more difficult to earn
   F. Use creative reinforcers, such as dropping quarters in a bank, putting money away for each goal reached, and ear-marked for something desirable. Take money back as a punishment if the goal is not reached.

Fig. 5-1. (Continued)

than out for pizza). Breaking response chains and preplanning behavior are other strategies.[13]

Some antecedents may be controlled by preplanning. Preplanning meals and snacks and having only proper foods in the house is preferable to expecting self-control when hungry. Preplanning social occasions and exercises is also helpful. Small portions of favorite foods may need to be included in the diet to avoid feelings of total deprivation and potential abandonment of dietary changes. Doing the right thing is enhanced by stimulus control. The goal is to decrease the number of times the person is exposed to tempting situations so that self-control is tested as rarely as possible.[14]

In some instances, responses occur in chains in which each response produces the stimulus for the next response. An example of a chain would be feeling tired, looking at the clock, realizing that it is bedtime, turning off the television, going to the kitchen, getting a snack, eating the snack, feeling satisfied (reinforcer), and going to bed. The components of the chain should be identified, and then a break in the chain should be planned, such as adding 5 minutes of stretching exercises after turning off the television.

Behavior. After identifying antecedents, one should explore the eating behavior itself, investigating the speed of eating, the presence of others, and activities carried on during meals or snacks, such as watching television. Breaking a chain of eating too rapidly, for example, is accomplished by introducing delays in eating. Members of the "clean plate club" need to leave some food on the plate. Concentrating on the act of eating and enjoying the flavors of the foods are recommended.

Consequences. Consequences of eating are described as reinforcements or rewards. According to Stunkard, "Since behavior is believed to be maintained by its consequences, efforts are made to arrange consequences that will maintain desirable behaviors, such as adherence to the weight control program."[1] The consequences of eating may be positive, negative, or neutral. In general, positive consequences are more effective in promoting change than negative or punishing consequences. Alternatives to eating may be included, such as walking or exercising, writing a letter, cleaning a part of the house, engaging in a hobby, and so on. One recommendation related to sodium restriction was for the client to set aside a quarter (or dollar) as a reward for using a spice or flavoring in place of salt.[11]

The client's current eating habits are pleasurable, and if food is considered its own reward, then new and different rewards must be established. Eating is a powerfully motivated behavior the occurrence of which is necessary to maintain the homeostasis of the organism. Without food consumption, the organism dies, so that eating provides reinforcement of a powerful biological drive. The dietitian needs to identify new reinforcers with clients. To be self-reinforcing, eating changes should be pleasurable. If new patterns are a chore and are disliked, they will fail to provide self-reinforcement.

The counselor can work with the client to establish reinforcers. Activity reinforcers may be identified by asking, "What do you like to do with your leisure time?" Reinforcers may be walking; attending movies, plays, or sporting events; taking a bath; gardening; hobbies; playing cards; reading; or whatever the individual prefers. Social reinforcers may be found by asking, "Whom do you like to be with?" Reinforcers may include visiting or phoning family or friends. Other questions are, "What do you find enjoyable?" and "What do you like to buy when you have extra money (other than inappropriate foods, of course)?"[14]

The counselor is also part of the reinforcement, and rather than focusing on failures, he should emphasize what the person has done right by providing verbal reward and praise. Remind the client to reward himself cognitively by telling himself he is making progress and has done something right. For the obese, the ability to fit into smaller-sized clothes hanging in the closet and the weight loss itself are reinforcing. New reinforcers, such as enjoyable activities, need to be established and introduced for weight maintenance, however. The reinforcement provided by significant others and self-monitoring are discussed later in the chapter.

After one or two eating changes or goals are identified, a schedule of reinforcement needs to be discussed and established. The schedule specifies which behaviors, if any, will be reinforced and how frequently reinforcement will be provided. Continuous reinforcement is the simplest method, but this may lose its effectiveness if used excessively. An alternative is intermittent reinforcement, such as reinforcement three times a day, or once a day. Eventually, the time between reinforcements may be lengthened. The schedule should be appropriate to the behavior one is trying to strengthen, convenient for the person to apply, and applied immediately for the greatest effect. Never reinforcing a behavior leads to its extinction.[15]

In some cases, contracts may be desirable. Contracts are clear statements of target behaviors of the individual; they specify the type of reinforcers to be used, the person who will deliver the reinforcers, and the frequency of reinforcement. They are signed and dated by the counselor and the client. Contracts ensure that all parties agree on the goals and procedures, and they provide a measurement of how close the client is to reaching his goals. The signatures help to ensure that the contract will be followed, since signing is a commitment and may provide added motivation to change.[11]

Completion of behavioral assessment is needed prior to counseling. Examination of the ABCs by the dietitian and the client assists both parties in understanding current eating behaviors and allows discussion of what can be changed. The role of the dietitian is to provide an integrated plan for the total nutrition program of each client. The dietitian serves as a guide or facilitator of change, rather than a director or controller of change, by suggesting behavioral techniques that are appropriate to the situation. The counselor should assist the client in learning to analyze this own eating problems and should suggest possible goals, strategies, and techniques to deal with them.

Since the client is not in daily contact with the counselor (unless the telephone is used for follow-up), he must be ready to assume personal responsibility for sound dietary changes, and must eventually become independent. He must learn to analyze and solve his own eating behavior problems. Have the client start with small, easy changes, which are most likely to be successful, and progress incrementally to more difficult ones in later sessions. To be self-reinforcing, the eating changes should be pleasurable ones. If the client enjoys potato chips, ice cream, pizza, and beer, he must find substitutes he enjoys, such as crisp apples, fresh grapes, unbuttered popcorn, and dietetic beverages. It may be sufficient to start by reducing the quantity of favorite foods consumed. Strategies must be highly individualized, and what is appropriate for one client may be inappropriate for another.

The client should be told to expect problems and some inappropriate eating binges, especially when he is under physical or emotional stress. Expecting total control over change is unrealistic and may lead to diminished self-esteem in clients who have problems following diets, with eventual abandonment of the dietary changes. Learning any new skill requires practice over a period of time. Repetition of the same new behaviors gradually becomes reinforcing. Support and forgiveness should be provided during any lapses. Enthusiasm for change may be expected to drop rapidly after the initial period, especially if frustration and disappointments arise, and weekly appointments with the counselor are needed in the beginning.

SELF-MONITORING

Self-monitoring, or keeping records of eating behaviors to be controlled, was intended originally as a means of supplying the counselor and client with data for analysis. The client records what, where, when, and how much he eats; the circumstances (e.g., watching television or feeling bored); and the persons present. The exercise of keeping records, however, was determined to have additional value of its own. It increased client awareness and understanding of current eating behaviors and the influences on them, and led to such realizations as "I'm eating too much during evening hours while I read." Data provided a basis for setting goals for change ("I'll eat a low calorie snack instead") and finding ways to reinforce new behaviors ("I'll tell myself how well I'm doing"). Keeping records served as a measure of the individual's commitment to change.[1] Weight loss graphs for the obese and records of physical exercise, blood sugar, and blood pressure are other self-monitoring techniques.

SELF-MANAGEMENT

In most behavior modification programs for weight control, the client and counselor are together only for brief durations and at specified intervals. Consequently, it is not possible for the counselor to be continually in control of the dispensing of rewards and punishments, or the withholding of rewards, for appropriate and inappropriate behavior, which is the basis of behavior modification. Therefore, self-regulation or self-management techniques are taught to the client so that he can regulate and control his own behavior. In this way, progress may be achieved in the intervals between meetings of the client and counselor.

Research has shown the importance of developing behavioral self-management techniques. Skinner explained that self-management, or "self-control," occurs when the individual manipulates the variables on which the behavior depends.[16] Self-management programs have been "designed to help persons become aware of and modify the social and physical antecedents of eating, to self-administer rewarding consequences for habit change [or appropriate behavior], or to self-administer aversive stimulation for inappropriate eating [behavior]."[10] As self-management programs have evolved, more emphasis has been placed on cognitive change. People have been helped to modify thought and beliefs that interfered with adherence to specific dietary regimes and to use self-reinforcing thoughts when appropriate behaviors occur.

Atkinson, Atkinson, and Hilgard have presented a program illustrating the use of learning principles for the self-regulation of food intake.[17] This program is based in part on the work of Stuart and Davis, and on that of O'Leary and Wilson.[18,19] The five-principle program is presented in Figure 5-2 as an example of the type of program used in self-regulation of eating.

SOCIAL SUPPORT

The client's environment includes a number of people he contacts daily. It is important to consider the person's family and significant others when planning lifestyle and dietary changes. The dietitian should include family members in counseling whenever possible, since the changes in food plans at home may affect them as well. Social factors may be contributing factors to obesity. If the family system supports an obese lifestyle, with high-calorie foods and little physical activity, change will be difficult for the client unless the whole family participates in the challenge.[11] There have also been suggestions that the involvement and support of spouse and family play an important role in weight loss.[20]

Ideally, family and friends are supportive of the efforts of the client in changing eating behaviors. The dietitian may need to discuss with clients the important role of support in achieving permanent change. In nonsupportive environments, the dietitian may suggest that the client request help from his family or friends by seeking their agreements not to eat forbidden foods in front of him, or not to purchase or prepare the wrong foods. In addition, the client might ask his spouse, family, and friends to offer positive reinforcement for his

SELF-MONITORING

Daily Log. Keep a detailed record of everything you eat. Note amount eaten, type of food and caloric value, time of day, and the circumstances of eating. This record will establish the caloric intake that is maintaining your present weight. It will also help to identify the stimuli that elicit and reinforce your eating behavior.

Weight Chart. Decide how much you want to lose and set a weekly goal for weight loss. Your weekly goal should be realistic (between 1 and 2 pounds). Record your weight each day on graph paper. In addition to showing how your weight varies with food intake, this visual record will reinforce your dieting efforts as you observe progress toward your goal.

CONTROLLING STIMULUS CONDITIONS

Use these procedures to narrow the range of stimuli associated with eating:
1 Eat only at predetermined times, at a specific table, using a special place mat, napkin, dishes, and so forth. Do *not* eat at other times or in other places (for example, while standing in the kitchen).
2 Do *not* combine eating with other activities, such as reading or watching television.
3 Keep in the house only those foods that are permitted on your diet.
4 Shop for food only after having had a full meal, buy only those items that are on a previously prepared list.

MODIFYING ACTUAL EATING BEHAVIOR

Use these procedures to break the chain of responses that make eating automatic:
1 Eat very slowly, paying close attention to the food.
2 Finish chewing and swallowing before putting more food on the fork.
3 Put your utensils down for periodic short breaks before continuing to eat.

DEVELOPING INCOMPATIBLE RESPONSES

When tempted to eat at times other than those specified, find a substitute activity that is incompatible with eating. For example, exercise to music, go for a walk, talk with a friend (preferably one who knows you are dieting), study your diet plan and weight graph, noting how much weight you have lost.

SELF-REINFORCEMENT

Arrange to reward yourself with an activity you enjoy (watching television, reading, planning a new wardrobe, visiting a friend) when you have maintained appropriate eating behavior for a day. Plan larger rewards (for example, buying something you want) for a specified amount of weight loss. Self-punishment (other than forgoing a reward) is probably less effective because dieting is a fairly depressing business anyway. But you might decrease the frequency of binge eating by immediately reciting to yourself the aversive consequences or by looking at an unattractive picture of yourself in a bathing suit.

Fig. 5-2. Self-regulation of eating. The program illustrates the use of learning principles to help control food intake. (From Atkinson, R.S., Atkinson, R.C., and Hilgard, E.F.: Introduction to Psychology. 8th Edition. © 1983 by Harcourt Brace Jovanovich, Inc. Reproduced by permission of the publisher. Based in part on Stuart, R.B., and David, B.: Slim Chance in a Fat World. Champaign, IL, Research Press, 1972 with permission of the publisher; and O'Leary, K.D., and Wilson, G.T.: Behavior Therapy: Application and Outcome. Englewood Cliffs, NJ, Prentice-Hall, 1975, pp. 332-333. Reprinted by permission of Prentice-Hall, Englewood Cliffs, NJ.)

efforts. Role-playing some of these situations with the client may be helpful.

When family members are present at the counseling session, they should be asked to discuss ways that they can contribute to the client's lifestyle change. Reinforcing proper behavior by the use of praise is an example. Controlling antecedents by having proper foods available is of great assistance. Family and friends should avoid acting the role of judge. "You shouldn't eat that," "It's bad for you," and "I told you so" are not helpful remarks. Jealous and envious reactions may also be expected. "You've lost enough weight," "Just this once won't hurt your diet," and "Your skin is getting to look awful" are remarks that the client may need to tolerate or confront.

APPLICATIONS

Obesity

The most frequent application of behavioral principles and methods to the treatment of nutritional problems has been in the management of obesity. In 1959, Stunkard noted that traditional psychotherapeutic approaches to obesity, as well as medical and dietary approaches, had not produced positive results. He reported that "most obese persons will not stay in treatment for obesity. Of those who stay in treatment most will not lose weight and of those who do lose weight, most will regain it."[21]

There is some difference of opinion regarding the efficacy of behavior modification techniques developed for use in treating overweight clients. Brownell reports that behavior therapy is more effective than any other treatment with which is has been compared and is an essential part of any weight reduction program.[22] Coates noted that "behavior modification has prospered under the protective shield of an especially good press."[10] These two reports, while emphasizing differing evaluative statements regarding the outcomes of behavior modification, are not mutually exclusive, and both could indeed be accurate. Obesity is a complex state and is not treated easily. The obese may be overweight for a variety of reasons, only one of which may be improper eating behaviors.

The American College of Sports Medicine, in a position statement, stressed that lifelong weight control requires commitment, and understanding of one's eating habits, and a willingness to change them.[23] To change any behavior, motivation must be present, and this is particularly true in changing eating behaviors. There are several factors relevant to the prediction of success in weight control, one of which is motivation to reduce weight. Brownell has stressed the importance of screening patients adequately before the initiation of any weight control program. A behavioral test of motivation as a screening device has been suggested.[22] Requiring a fee for treatment is one approach, but a deposit-refund system has been used also. In the latter system, patients are asked to deposit money, which is later returned if the patient attends meetings faithfully and/or achieves a previously determined weight loss. This system appears to be effective in reducing the drop-out rate.

Eating Disorders

An early report detailed the use of behavior modification techniques for a different nutritional disorder, anorexia nervosa, a chronic failure to eat.[24] A female who was five feet four inches tall weighed only 47 pounds at the start of her behavior therapy. Before therapy commenced, the hospital environment provided many amenities and privileges. Because she appeared to enjoy them, these privileges and amenities were removed so that they could be used to reinforce appropriate behaviors, in this case, eating. All of the attention and sympathy that the hospital staff had used to coax the patient to eat were withdrawn. The therapist ate one meal a day with the patient, and the staff was allowed only to greet the patient on entering the room.

The social reinforcement that had helped to maintain non-eating behavior was withheld so that it could be used later to strengthen eating behaviors. The therapist talked to the patient to reinforce her behavior when she picked up her fork, lifted food toward her mouth, chewed food, or performed any other eating behavior. She was then allowed the use of a radio or television, but only after meals at which she increased her food intake over previous meals. As she gained strength and weight, other reinforcers were introduced, such as the privilege of choosing her own menu or inviting other patients to dine with her. Later reinforcers included walks, visitors, and mail.

The treatment was successful, and after 8 weeks of therapy, she was discharged to a program of outpatient follow-up, weighing 64 pounds. Five years later, she had maintained her weight between 78 and 80 pounds and was successfully employed.[25] Locating potential reinforcers or behavior strengtheners is an essential first step in any treatment program. What reinforces behavior for one person may not function as a reinforcer for another.

A later study reported the successful inpatient behavioral treatment of anorexia and bulimia.[26] The treatment program was associated with increases in body weight and caloric consumption, which were generally maintained at two-year follow-up. Self-monitoring of eating behavior, including caloric intake, emesis, and bulimia, proved to be a useful maintenance strategy. Other studies have noted the importance of self-monitoring and daily logging of intake, weight, and details of binge/purge episodes on progress and successful treatment of anorexia and bulimia.[27-29] These reported successes of behavioral treatment of anorexia and bulimia have involved inpatient therapy and outpatient follow-up.

Another finding from the research on anorexia nervosa concerns the effect of size of food portions on eating behavior. The serving of larger food portions was associated with increased food intake. Apparently, the subjects had been eating a relatively fixed proportion of the amount of food presented, whether the portion was large or small. This pattern of eating has been noted to occur in obese people as well, but not in normal adults or in young children.[8]

Behavior modification has also been used successfully in the treatment of chronic food refusal in handicapped children. Records of conditions before treatment began indicated that all patients accepted little food, expelled food frequently, and engaged in disruptive behavior. Treatment methods used were social praise, access to preferred foods, brief periods of play with toys, and forced feeding. Marked behavioral improvement was noted for each patient as well as an increase in the amount of food consumed. Further improvements were noted at 7- to 30-month follow-up.[30]

Diabetes Mellitus

Behavior modification methods have proven to be a useful component in the management of diabetes mellitus. Historically, poor patient adherence to dietary regimens has been a problem. Behavioral interventions such as cuing, self-monitoring, and reinforcement for appropriate behavior have been effective in promoting dietary adherence for patients with Type I diabetes. Success has not been as great, however, with behavioral techniques used in weight loss programs for obese patients with Type II diabetes.[31] As previously noted, though, the problem of controlling obesity from the standpoint of any particular treatment is complex.

Behavioral management techniques have also been used with young diabetic patients to improve their adherence to prescribed medical regimens. Subjects were given training in behavioral self-management. In addition, they received training in negotiation and contracting, which allowed them to develop a contract to earn reinforcement from parents for using learned self-management skills. These behavioral procedures led to a large increase in adherence to the prescribed medical regimen.[32] Young adults with diabetes improved their ability to estimate their blood glucose levels after participating in a discrimination training program, in which they received feedback regarding the accuracy of their estimates. These resulting increases in accuracy of glucose level estimation have established the opportunity for better nutritional control of the disease.[33]

Cardiovascular Diseases

In the Multiple Risk Factor Intervention Trial (MRFIT), behavioral scientists and nutritionists worked cooperatively with the aim of changing behaviors related to diet and smoking on a long-term basis to reduce the risk of cardiovascular disease. A self-evaluation system for monitoring food intake was developed so that the counselor could estimate the subject's progress in making appropriate dietary changes. A scoring system was used for classifying foods according to their fat and cholesterol content as well as their predicted effect on blood cholesterol. Subjects could use the system and select alternative food choices to meet appropriate eating goals. The self-monitoring records were employed as a method of measuring compliance, and also served to reinforce change and to provide positive feedback for appropriate behavior.[34]

In a study concering the dietary management of hypertension, Tillotson and co-workers identified steps in patients' behavior that were critical for the success of permanent dietary management.[35] These steps are as follows:

1. The person acknowledges that he has high blood pressure.
2. The person considers diet as a sole or adjunctive method of helping to control high blood pressure.
3. The person participates in assessing his current dietary pattern, social environment, thoughts, beliefs, and feelings.
4. The person acknowledges that successful dietary change will require an extended period of time.
5. The person participates in developing an overall strategy and in setting long-term goals for blood pressure and diet.
6. The person participates in planning each step of dietary change.
7. The person makes each dietary change.
8. The person participates in assessing whether he has succeeded in making each change.
9. The person participates in assessing his attainment of blood pressure control.
10. The person participates in devising a plan for maintaining dietary changes as goals are approached.

Personnel Management

The behavior of employees is of major concern to supervisors who are interested in both productivity and good human relations. Blanchard and Johnson's book *The One Minute Manager* provides examples of behavioral modification strategies.[2] Goals begin new behaviors, and in the "one minute goal," the manager uses observable, measurable behavioral terms to describe the discrepancy between the actual and desired performances. Because behaviors are believed to be maintained by their consequences, the "one minute praise" and the "one minute reprimand," examples of rewards and punishments, are recommended. While most supervisors attempt to catch subordinates doing things wrong, Blanchard and Johnson suggest that they notice employees doing something right or approximately right and then gradually move them toward the desired behavior. The one-minute praise is used immediately to reinforce proper behavior. Eventually, some employees begin to praise themselves for the proper behavior, which provides additional reinforcement. The one-minute reprimand is also used immediately and concentrates on the improper behavior, not on the person.

IMPLICATIONS FOR THERAPY

Brownell has pointed out two major advantages of behavior therapy. Attrition from treatment programs is low, and patients in behavior therapy programs seem to show improved psychological functioning. Brownell asserts that such improvement has important implications for compliance and motivation, ingredients ultimately important for any type of treatment regimen.[22]

While eating behavior patterns are not altered easily, behavior modification therapy offers promising techniques that may be helpful to both the client and the counselor. Analysis of the ABCs—the antecedents, behavior, and consequences of eating—by the counselor and client leads to an understanding of the problems, the setting of goals, and the development of strategies for change. Effort should be made to arrange consequences that reinforce and maintain desirable changes, with an ultimate goal being independent client self-management. Behavior modification may be used in conjunction with other counseling and education strategies.

SUGGESTED ACTIVITIES

1. Complete a food diary for 3 days. Identify the cues for eating and the reinforcers. Set one goal for change, and identify the particular reinforcers to be used.

2. Ask a friend or family member to keep a food record. Work with him to set one goal for change and identify the reinforcers. Follow up on his progress after one week.

3. Arrange to watch an adult interact with a child (or children) for half an hour. Tally the number of times the adult attends to the child's desirable behaviors, which reinforces them, versus the number of times desirable behaviors are ignored, which may lead to their extinction. Note whether the adult reinforces undesirable behaviors by responding to them.

4. Make a list of leisure time activities that you enjoy, people you like to be with, and things you would purchase with extra money, to identify your own reinforcers.

5. You have been assigned two chapters to read (or a paper to write) during the next few days. Select an appropriate reinforcer for yourself, and identify a time schedule for dispensing the reinforcer.

6. Select an excessive behavior of your own that you would like to diminish. For 3 days, record those situations in which it occurs. Identify the controlling stimulus just prior to the behavior, and identify the reinforcement.

7. Identify situations where modeling occurs.

8. In a social situation with friends, tally the number of times in one-half hour that you dispense social approval (smiles, nods, appreciative words) versus disapproval (frowns, disparaging words).

9. List ten phrases of social approval that you are comfortable using with others.

REFERENCES

1. Stunkard, A., and Berthold, H.: What is behavior therapy? Am. J. Clin. Nutr., *41*:821, 1985.
2. Blanchard, K., and Johnson, S.: The One Minute Manager. New York, Berkley Books, 1981.
3. Hill, W.F.: Principles of Learning. Palo Alto, CA, Mayfield Pub. Co., 1981.
4. Schwartz, B., and Lacey, H.: Behaviorism, Science and Human Nature. New York, W.W. Norton, 1982.
5. Sims, H.P., and Manz, C.C.: Modeling influences on employee behavior. Personnel J., *61*:58, 1982.
6. Bandura, A.: Social Learning Theory. Englewood Cliffs, NJ, Prentice-Hall, 1977.
7. Craighead, W.E., Kazdin, A.E., and Mahoney, M.J.: Behavior Modification. Boston, Houghton Mifflin, 1976.
8. Barlow, D.H., and Tillotson, J.L.: Behavioral science and nutrition: A new perspective. J. Am. Diet. Assoc., *72*:368, 1978.
9. Mahoney, M.J., and Caggiula, A.W.: Applying behavioral methods to nutritional counseling. J. Am. Diet. Assoc., *72*:372, 1978.
10. Coates, T.J.: Eating—A Psychological Dilemma. J. Nutr. Ed., *13*:S34, 1981.
11. Rabb, C., and Tillotson, J.L. (eds): Heart to Heart. Washington, DC, U.S. Dept. of Health and Human Services, 1983.
12. Fensterheim, H., and Baer, J.: Don't Say Yes When You Want to Say No. New York, Dell, 1975.
13. Building Nutrition Counseling Skills. Vol. II. Washington, DC, U.S. Dept. of Health and Human Services, 1984.
14. Storlie, J., and Jordan, H.A.: Behavioral Management of Obesity. New York, Spectrum Pub., 1984.
15. Martin, G., and Pear, J.: Behavior Modification. Englewood Cliffs, NJ, Prentice-Hall, 1978.
16. Skinner, B.F.: Science and Human Behavior. New York, Macmillan, 1953.
17. Atkinson, R.L., Atkinson, R.C., and Hilgard, E.: Introduction to Psychology. 8th ed. New York, Harcourt Brace Jovanovich, 1983.
18. Stuart, R.B., and Davis, B.: Slim Chance in a Fat World, Champaign, IL, Research Press, 1972.
19. O'Leary, K., and Wilson, G.: Behavior Therapy: Applications and Outcome. Englewood Cliffs, NJ, Prentice-Hall, 1975.
20. Abrahamson, E.: Behavioral treatment of obesity. Behav. Therapist, *6*:103, 1983.

21. Stunkard, A., and McLaren-Hume, M.: The results of treatment for obesity. Arch. Intern. Med., *103*:79, 1959.
22. Brownell, K.: The psychology and physiology of obesity. J. Am. Diet. Assoc., *84*:406, 1984.
23. American College of Sports Medicine: Position statement on proper and improper weight loss programs. Med. and Sci. in Sports and Exercise, *15*:IX, 1983.
24. Bachrach, A., Erwin, W., and Mohr, J.: The control of eating behavior in an anorexic by operant conditioning techniques. *In* Case Studies in Behavior Modification. Edited by L. Ullman and L.P. Krasner. New York, Holt, Rinehart, and Winston, 1965.
25. Reese, E.: The Analysis of Human Operant Behavior. Dubuque, IA, William C. Brown Co., 1966.
26. Cinciripini, P., Kornblith, S., Turner, S., and Hersen, M.: A behavioral program for the management of anorexia and bulimia. J. Nerv. Ment. Dis., *171*:186, 1983.
27. Leitenberg, H., Gross, J., Peterson, J., and Rosen, J.: Analysis of an anxiety model and the process of change during exposure plus response prevention treatment of bulimia nervosa. Behav. Therapy, *15*:3, 1984.
28. Cullari, S., and Redmon, W.: Treatment of bulimorexia through behavior therapy and diet modification. Behav. Therapist, *6*:165, 1983.
29. Smith, G., and Medlik, L.: Modification of binge eating in anorexia nervosa. Behav. Psychotherapy, *11*:249, 1983.
30. Riordan, M.M., et al.: Behavioral assessment and treatment of chronic food refusal in handicapped children. J. Appl. Behav. Anal., *17*:327, 1984.
31. Wing, R., Epstein, L., and Norwalk, M.: Dietary adherence in patients with diabetes. Behav. Med. Update, *6*:17, 1984.
32. Gross, A.: Self-management training and medication compliance in children with diabetes. Child Fam. Behav. Ther., *4*:47, 1982.
33. Gross, A.: Discrimination of blood glucose levels in insulin-dependent diabetics. Behav. Modification, *7*:369, 1983.
34. Remmell, P.S., Gorder, D.D., Hall, Y., and Tillotson, J.L.: Assessing dietary adherence in the Multiple Risk Factor Intervention Trial (MRFIT). J. Am. Diet. Assoc., *76*:351, 1980.
35. Tillotson, J.L. Winston, M.C., and Hall, Y.: Critical behaviors in the dietary management of hypertension. J. Am. Diet. Assoc., *84*:290, 1984.

6

Group Process

When people gather together in groups, they do not act in the same way as when they are alone or with one other person. This "behavior" that is observed when people come together is often discussed under the topic of "group dynamics." Each group develops its own pattern of interaction as it goes through various phases, and as members become comfortable in the group, learning to know and trust one another. The individual who is promoted into management is often expected to convert his behavior from performing a task to managing a staff without being given the necessary training to exercise the required new skills. Activities such as conducting performance appraisals, counseling and disciplining staff, and facilitating group meetings require well-honed communication skills. When people are advanced into management without adequate training in these areas, the chances of their succeeding as administrators are hindered.

This chapter provides the dietitian with a general overview of the dynamics inherent in groups and the variables that influence their direction, growth, and development. These process variables refer to how the group functions internally, how the members relate to each other and the procedures they follow, how they communicate among themselves, and how they do their work as a group.[1] The following topics are discussed: the value in understanding the group's dynamics as an aid to solving problems, the responsibilities and roles of facilitators and participants, the guidelines for managing meetings effectively, and the uses and value of groups as a tool in nutritional counseling.

Much of this chapter is devoted to exploring skills of the group leader and participants. The reader is cautioned, however, that one cannot develop these skills simply from reading a chapter, or even from reading it again and again. To develop these skills, a person must make a personal commitment to risk feeling unsure and awkward as he attempts to practice them. An individual need not wait until he is in a management position. In fact, the time to develop group skills is while one is still a student or a subordinate. The skills can be practiced with friends, with family, and in the community.

In that way, when one graduates to a position of authority, the skills will have become refined from the earlier practice and experience.

Group skills help the dietitian to manage change with both staff and client groups. Ongoing change in organizations is inevitable. When changes are minor, the administrator can simply announce the changes and expect others to follow without resistance; however, other changes may be perceived as threatening by the staff. When changes arouse a sense of fear, ambiguity, and uncertainty, they are resisted.

There is a direct correlation between the amount of time, consideration, and participation in the proposed change allotted to those affected by the change and the amount of resistance likely to occur. When people are given consideration and an opportunity to voice their anxieties and questions, with their recommendations being incorporated whenever possible, they are less likely to resist the changes and more likely to assist in upholding them among others who may resist. When an entire work group is involved in discussion of problems and potential changes, with their supervisor acting as facilitator, agreement can be reached to employ new methods, procedures, or solutions. Those members of the group who later object are reminded by the others that they had adequate opportunity to make suggestions and express their concerns, and that objecting now is inappropriate.

Group skills are invaluable for solving problems. When managed correctly, groups have the potential to arrive at solutions that are superior to those that might arise from one-to-one counseling. This phenomenon is called "synergy" and is discussed in detail later in the chapter.

Groups skills are an asset in nutritional counseling as well. They allow counselees to experience and express mutual support and reinforcement, to share in adapting creative solutions to problems that others may have solved and to use group methods such as brainstorming and role-playing to develop and "try out" new behavior. Rehearsing new behavior for the real world is known to be one of the most effective strategies for change.[2] Group counseling and individual counseling may be used together. Specific or unique problems are best handled individually with the dietitian. Holding a group session is the most efficient way to give information to several people who may have similar concerns or problems. The final section of this chapter discusses nutritional counseling.

Dietitians need to be aware of the inherent power and influence of the informal work group. Since the 1920s, when the Hawthorne studies were carried out at the Western Electric plant near Chicago, social scientists have been studying the "Hawthorne effect," which refers to the theory, and its corollaries, that employees perform more efficiently when they believe that they are being given special attention. The theory suggests that the major influences affecting efficiency and production are group social structures, group norms, and group pressures.

The administrative dietitian needs to be sensitive to the dynamics and influences of the informal work group. He must learn ways to provide a forum where social, task-related, and organizational concerns can be expressed, responses can be offered, and any resistance to change can be overcome. To become conscious of the influence inherent in the informal work group, and to tap into the grapevine of informal communication, the administrative dietitian needs to be aware of the networks of communication that exist within the department as well as those within the organization.

Communication networks are the patterns of message flow, or linkages of who actually speaks to whom.[1] In all organizations, there are distinctions between the "permissible" and the actual channels of communication and network linkages. The permissible channels are the linkages dictated by the organizational structure, which determines the hierarchy of power and influence; the actual channels are the patterns that actually occur. Often, secretaries are ultimately more influential, because of their connections within the network, than others who are considerably higher on the organizational flow chart. A later section in the chapter discusses "process meetings" as a way of tapping into the informal group and airing common group concerns.

Although they constitute a minority in the 1980s, some people perform best when under the direction of an authoritarian leader. When someone has come from a background where he has not been encouraged to think and has been punished for initiating ideas, it is predictable that in a work situation he will lack the self-confidence to offer suggestions within a group. If he is treated with patience, however, and is given continued positive reinforcement each time he risks contributing an idea, he may gradually gain the confidence to become a valuable group member. In general, however, members of today's work force perform best in groups with a leader who can act as a facilitator, involving employees rather than prescribing to them. A "facilitator" is one who understands the value of group decision-making, and sees his functions as being to help the group get started, to establish a climate of work, to give support to others, and to keep the group on track so that its objectives are achieved. The group's activities and the facilitator's attitude toward the group are based on respect for what can be accomplished through group discussion and on the fostering of a group climate where people feel comfortable and secure enough to contribute their ideas.

Although interpersonal and group interaction skills can be taught, the most effective way for individuals to learn them is through experiencing and observing others whom they admire and view as effective communicators. Communication skills can be effectively "caught" as well as taught, and the dietitian has an opportunity to develop these skills in his staff and clients through his own "modeling" of them. Whether or not he intends it, and whether his behavior is good or bad, the dietitian is a role model to his staff and clients. By learning interpersonal and group skills and then consciously applying them, the dietitian constructively and proactively enhances their development among staff and clients.

FACILITATOR PREPARATION

The facilitator's responsibilities begin prior to the discussion, in his preparation of the appropriate meeting environment. He must make sure that the room itself is comfortable, with adequate ventilation and lighting, and with a consciously arranged seating pattern. Sitting in a circle, for example, allows group members to see one another's faces, which tends to increase interaction among them. When people are arranged at long rectangular tables, each person tends to interact most with those in direct view and little with those on either side of him.[3]

When meetings involve individuals who do not know one another, the facilitator should supply name tags or cards for everyone in the group. A sense of group spirit develops more quickly when people use one another's names as they interact.[3] Allowing members time to introduce themselves is time well spent toward developing a comfortable climate. "Small talk" in groups is not a small matter. Just hearing one another allows the members to make some assumptions that help them to reduce anxiety. An individual's tone of voice, dress, diction, and manner provide valuable clues to his character. Often, negative inferences disappear after the other's voice is heard and some information regarding his background is gathered.

GROUP FACILITATION SKILLS

The dietetic literature emphasizes the needs of nutrition counselors and educators to assist in group problem solving by further developing their roles as experts, information disseminators, diagnosticians, team members, emphathizers, and group facilitators.[4,5] Most dietitians will eventually need to direct others in groups and facilitate interaction among them. Effective facilitation requires training and discipline to stay in the role of guide and not become a participant. Described in the following paragraphs are specific skills that need to be practiced as one trains to develop group facilitation skills.[1,3,6]

Relieving Social Concerns. A tenet of group dynamics suggests that social concerns take precedence over "task" or work-related concerns. In other words, an individual's first concern is with being accepted and acknowledged as worthy. If he feels anxiety about being with unknown others, or others who may bear him ill will, he generally will not participate. One way a facilitator can attend to social concerns is to spend a few minutes at the beginning of each meeting, allowing people to interact socially and to reestablish positive regard for one another. If ill will does exist among some of the participants, and the facilitator is aware of it, he can attempt to have the members resolve their conflict prior to the meeting, or if they are willing, he can assist them in resolving the conflict at the meeting. Only after the members have had their social concerns met can they wholeheartedly participate in "task" concerns.

Tolerating Silence. After the facilitator has made his opening remarks, has made sure that everyone knows everyone else, has articulated the desire for everyone's participation, and has stated the reasons or purpose for the meeting, he might rephrase the topic in the form of a question and then invite someone to comment. Because members are frequently hesitant to express opinions with which their superior may disagree, they often wait to hear his opinion first. There may be times when no one wants to initiate discussion and the group sits in silence, waiting for the facilitator to save them and reduce the tension. Silence is likely to occur most during the early stages of an ongoing group. Once the group comes to understand that the facilitator truly does not intend to dominate, lead, or force his opinion, members will begin to use the meeting time to interact with one another. For those first few meetings, however, the facilitator should repeat his intention not to participate, should encourage others to participate, and then should just sit patiently. If he tolerates the silence long enough, someone will eventually take the responsibility for directing the discussion.

Guiding Unobtrusively and Encouraging Interaction. The facilitator guides indirectly, helping the members to relate better to one another and to complete the task. He does not allow himself to become the focus. The facilitator can encourage interaction among the group members rather than with himself by looking away from speakers in the group as they attempt to harness his eyes. Although this behavior may seem rude, the speaker will quickly get the idea and look to the other group members for feedback and response as he continues to talk. Another way to keep the group's attention off himself is for the facilitator to resist the temptation to make a reply after others talk. He needs to wait for someone else to reply. If no one else makes a comment, however, the facilitator can ask for reactions. A question such as "Any reaction to that?" is preferred to "my reaction is . . . ."

Because the facilitator wishes to keep the focus off himself and on the group, he should remind group members during the first few minutes of the meeting that he sees his purpose primarily as getting things started and then simply serving as a guide. This assertion will eventually be tested. Most people have heard that same sentiment expressed by teachers and others, and have learned that while some of them do mean it, the majority are paying it lip service only, want things done their way, and expect ultimately to be followed.

Knowing When and How to Resume Control. Just as a facilitator who rules and dominates in an authoritarian manner can stifle the group's creativity, facilitators who are too timid, uncertain, or frightened, and who let the group wander, can hinder the group's potential for synergy, i.e., for finding superior solutions. Facilitators need to determine if the group is capable of facilitating for itself. When it is, the facilitator's function is to remain on the sidelines. Only when there are no competent participants available to perform the necessary functions does the facilitator become an active member of the group.

Reinforcing Multi-Sided Nature of Discussion. The facilitator can reinforce the nondogmatic, multi-sided nature of discussion by phrasing questions so that they are open-ended. Examples include questions such as "How do you feel about that?" "Who in your opinion...?" and "What would be some way to...?" Facilitators need to think before asking questions in order to avoid closed and leading questions, questions that can be answered by only one or two words, or questions suggesting a limited number of alternative responses.

Exercising Control Over Talkative Participants. The most common problem facilitators have is knowing what to say to someone who is overly talkative. There are, of course, many appropriate ways of handling this participant, and individual facilitators need to decide which techniques they personally feel most comfortable using, keeping in mind that when they interact with any single member of the group, all other participants experience the interaction vicariously. If the facilitator treats individual participants without respect, or humiliates or embarrasses them, all members will be affected by the experience.

Several techniques can be effective in dealing with the talkative participant. The facilitator might interrupt the participant, commenting that his point has been understood, and begin immediately to paraphrase concisely so that the participant knows that he has been understood. While it is true that some group members talk excessively because they enjoy talking and because they believe that they are raising their status within the group through the quantity of their interaction, other talkative members often repeat themselves because of insecurity. They are not convinced that they have been understood. Usually, this kind of participant stops talking after being paraphrased. Of course, this process may need to be repeated several times during the course of the discussion.

A second problem arises with the participant who simply enjoys talking and does perceive increased status from it. This person does not stop talking after being paraphrased. He may need to be told that short concise statements are easier to follow and that the group is losing the point from his extensive commentary. If that does not work, the facilitator may need to talk with the participant privately. Often, a talkative group member is unaware that others are offended by his domination. The facilitator can point out to him that he has noticed others stirring and wanting to enter the discussion. It needs to be stressed to these participants that long-windedness cuts down on the time allowed for others to contribute to the discussion.

Encouraging Silent Members. For various reasons, including boredom, indifference, felt superiority, timidity, and insecurity, there are usually some members who refuse to participate. The facilitator's action toward them depends on what is causing them to be silent. The facilitator can arouse interest by asking for the opinions of silent members. The person sitting next to him can be questioned, and then the silent member can be asked for his opinion of what his colleague has said. If the silence stems from insecurity, the best method is to reinforce positively each attempt at interjection. A smile, a nod, or a comment of appreciation for his opinion is sufficient. Sometimes silent members "shout out" nonverbal signals. An overt frown, nod, and/or pounding fingers are all signals that the individual has strong feelings. These overt, nonverbal signals should be interpreted as the silent member's willingness to be called upon to elaborate; however, if the silent member has his head down and has a blank facial expression, it would be a mistake to force the individual into the discussion.

Halting Side Conversations. Generally, the facilitator should not embarrass members who are engaged in private conversations by drawing attention to them in the presence of the group. Their conversation may be related to the subject, or it may be personal. If the side conversation becomes distracting to other members of the group, those engaged in the conversation might be called by name and asked an easy question.

Discouraging Wisecracks. If someone in the group disrupts with too much humor or too many wisecracks, the facilitator needs to determine at what point the humor stops being a device to relieve tension in the group and starts to interfere with the group's interests. When the facilitator believes that the humor is taking the focus off group issues and onto the joker, he needs to interrupt, smiling, with a comment such as "Now let's get down to business." If the comment needs to be made a second time, intense eye contact with the joker and no smile as the same remark is repeated usually halts the disruption.

Helping the Group to Stay on the Topic. When the group itself seems unable to stick to the agenda and wanders, a device under used by facilitators is a flip chart to jot down points that have been agreed upon as a way to chart the group's progress. With a minimum of interaction, the facilitator can prod the group on by simply summarizing and writing down the points. Generally, the group's reaction is to go on to the next item on the agenda.

Avoiding Acknowledgment of the Facilitator's Preferences. The facilitator hinders the group when he praises the ideas he likes and belittles those he dislikes. It is particularly important that he avoid making comments that may be taken as disapproval, condescension, sarcasm, personal cross-examination, or self-approval. Once the group members know the facilitator's preferences, they will tend to incorporate these preferences in their own comments. Because the administrative dietitian is in a position to reward or punish subordinates, the group members quickly learn that if what the supervisor wants is to be followed and not disagreed with, that is how they must behave toward him.

FACILITATOR/PARTICIPANT FUNCTIONS

In addition to the specific skills requried of facilitators, there are numerous group skills that both participants and facilitators should possess. There is a mistaken notion that it is the facilitator's responsibility alone to see to it that the group's tasks are accomplished and that a healthy group spirit is maintained. In reality, these responsibilities belong to anyone who has the training and insight to diagnose the group's weaknesses and who has the skills to correct them. Because most people are used to being "led" in groups, the facilitator may need to reinforce verbally the functions that all participants are expected to perform. The following paragraphs describe some of the skills or functions that both facilitators and participants have a mutual obligation to develop in themselves:[7]

1. Groups need members to propose new ideas, goals, and procedures. Individual members are expected to accept the responsibility of *initiating*. Any member who has the insight into what should be initiated and waits for someone else to do it is ignoring an obligation.

2. Everyone shares the responsibility of *seeking information and opinions*. One does not have to have great knowledge of the topic being discussed to be a valuable member. Asking the right questions and seeking information from others in the group who have knowledge are valuable functions.

3. *Clarifying* what others have said by adding examples, illustrations, or explanations is a major contribution. We are not all on the same "wavelength." Because of background, life experiences, education, natural intelligence, or environment, some people tend to

understand one another more easily than others do. Two people who have grown up under similar conditions, for example, have an easier time communicating than two people from different backgrounds. If one understands what someone else in the group is struggling to make clear and adds examples and explanations to clarify the thought for the others, he has made a significant contribution. Simply nodding in agreement and saying nothing is a disservice to the others.

4. Another function related to clarifying is *coordinating* relationships among facts, ideas, and suggestions. If one has the insight to understand how the ideas and activities of two or more group members are related and how they can be coordinated, the member serves a valuable function in expressing this relationship to the others.

5. *Orienting* is a name given to the function of processing for the group the pattern of its interaction and progress. The orienter clarifies the group's purpose or goal, defines the position of the group, and summarizes or suggests the direction of the discussion. Orienting by providing frequent internal summaries, for example, allows the group an opportunity to verify whether everyone is understanding the direction in which the group is going, and provides those who disagree or who have misunderstood with the opportunity to speak.

6. Perhaps the least understood and most valuable function one can perform for a group is *being a supporter*. A supporter is one who praises, agrees, indicates warmth and solidarity, and verbally indicates to the others that he is in agreement with what is being proposed. It is a valuable function because without verbal support from others, good ideas and suggestions are often disregarded. If one person expresses an idea that the majority dislike and that no one supports, the idea is quickly dismissed. Generally, if only one other person supports the idea, the group will seriously consider the proposal. Frequently, a minority opinion can gain majority support because a single supporter agrees, causing the group to consider seriously the possible merits of the proposal. Support can be given by briefly remarking, "I agree," "Well said," "I wish I had said that," or "Those are my sentiments, too." Generally, one person alone cannot influence a group; one person with a supporter, however, has an excellent chance of doing so.

7. *Harmonizing* is also a valuable contribution to the group. It includes mediating differences between others, reconciling disagreement, and bringing about collaboration from conflict. It is common for individuals to sit silently as they hear the valid arguments on both sides of an issue. One of the ways in which discussion differs from debate, however, is that discussion assumes that most issues are multi-sided while debate tends to lend itself to two-sided

issues only. The group member who verbally reinforces the positive aspects of the various factions and helps to suggest new and alternative solutions that include the best points of all sides is harmonizing.

8. Conflict, stress, and tension in groups is inevitable. When the stress or the tension mounts, it can enhance the conflict and the disagreement. Individuals who can find humor in the situation, reduce the formality or status differences among group members, and relax the others are called "tension relievers." A problem can occur when the tension reliever seeks recognition for himself and continues to joke, drawing the attention away from the issues. *Relieving tension* is valuable up to a point, after which it can be disruptive.

9. The final function in this discussion is *gatekeeping*. In gatekeeping, one notices which members have been sending out signals that they want to speak but have not had the courage or opportunity to enter the discussion. Gatekeeping ensures that all have an equal chance to be heard. As pointed out in the discussion of the facilitator's functions, there is a difference between people who are nonverbally signaling that they have strong feelings—by raising their eyebrows, tapping loudly, or grunting—and people who are silent, have their heads down and are maintaining a neutral expression. Group members become uncomfortable when they sense that other members might force them to talk. All members share the responsibility to protect others from being coerced into sharing opinions. Gatekeepers tend to say things such as "You look like you have strong feelings,"or "I can tell by your face that you disapprove." Such comments are generally all the prodding the silent participant needs to enter the discussion.

Too often individuals believe that in the ideal group, a single leader is responsible for each of the functions just discussed. In fact, all members—participants as well as facilitators—are responsible, and they need to be alert to perform as many of the functions as they see a need for. Some people may be natural "harmonizers" or natural "orienters," or may be able to perform effortlessly some other valuable function; however, if the group needs a gatekeeper and none is present, the natural harmonizer who sees the need must exercise the gatekeeping function. One of the ways people familiar with group dynamics and with the skills needed to enhance the workings of groups can detect members who have had training in the same area is by their willingness to act on their insight to correct a weakness in the group. As pointed out in a previous chapter, the mind operates several times as fast as the speed of human speech. While members of the group are talking, other sophisticated group members need to be reflecting on the dynamics of the group and on its needs at the moment. This process leads to an understanding of which functions need to be performed to help the group accomplish its task and maintain its healthy spirit.

Paradox of Group Dynamics. There is a paradox inherent in groups: They possess the potential, on the one hand, to stimulate creative thinking and to promote a decision or solution that is superior to what any individual working alone could accomplish. On the other hand, groups possess the potential to stifle creative thinking and thus promote a quality of outcome inferior to what individuals working alone might accomplish. Ordinarily, no one person is solely responsible for what happens in any given session; however, whether a group becomes a force to promote creative thinking and problem solving or a force that inhibits these functions depends primarily on the skills of its leader, and to a lesser degree, on the skills of the participants. There are specific behavior patterns that help a group to function effectively, and others that hinder the progress. Knowing how to facilitate positive behavior in groups and how to inhibit the negative behavior is an asset to dietitians.

SYNERGY

The dietitian needs to appreciate "group process" and to discover what can be done to stimulate his work and/or client group so that it becomes a creative force that promotes "synergy." Synergy refers to the phenomenon that the group's product (i.e., conclusion, solution, or decision) is qualitatively and/or quantitatively superior to what the most resourceful individual within the group could have produced by working alone.[8] Today, much is understood about the phenomenon; however, it has not yet filtered into management practice. Although greatly influenced by the style of their facilitators, all groups possess the potential to be either a force for creative innovative thinking or a force that works to preserve the status quo and stifle new ideas. The purpose of this section is to make the dietitian aware of the principles regarding synergy and to provide suggestions on how to apply them. The major variables that affect the group's potential for synergy are whether a single expert is available within the group, whether the group is heterogeneous or homogeneous, and whether the group and its facilitator are trained in the consensus-seeking process.

The facilitator should begin each meeting by stating his desire to promote a climate of acceptance and freedom of expression. Hearing the facilitator express this desire helps to set a group "norm" whereby everyone has a responsibility to participate. A norm is an unwritten rule to which the group adheres. Members "pick up" the code of appropriate behavior by noticing what the facilitator reinforces positively, ignores, tolerates, or rejects. The facilitator's expressing the desire for everyone to participate and the right of each member to express subjective opinions without being abused by others will eventually be tested. It is not enough to articulate these norms; they must be enforced. If individuals are abused by others, told to be silent, embarrassed, humiliated, or insulted, for example, and the facilitator doesn't intervene to protect them, his articulated norm will be discounted and the actual behavior that has been tolerated will be considered the "real" norm. For that reason, it is critical that group facilitators realize the importance of their function to stimulate group interaction while protecting group members from being verbally abused or stifled. Realizing that synergy is most likely to occur in groups where people can react authentically and are free to challenge the facilitator and the other participants, the administrative dietitian needs to convince the group that they need to listen and respond honestly to one another's ideas.

As a rule, if a single expert is available and the rest of the group members are relatively ignorant of the matter being discussed, the expert should make the decision. In practice, however, there is usually no single expert available, and some group members are more informed than others, with a wide range of opinions being represented in the group. Under those conditions, the potential for synergy exists.

The variable of a heterogeneous versus homogeneous group of participants is more complicated. When group members are untrained in the consensus-seeking process and form a homogeneous group, they have less conflict and generally produce superior decisions to those produced by an untrained heterogeneous group. It is understandable that people who are similar in age, background, culture, life experiences, values, and the like have an easier time agreeing than those with whom they have little in common.

The heterogeneous group that is untrained is likely to respond in one of the following ways. If individuals in the group do not know one another, they will probably remain silent. Most people become anxious in the presence of strangers, whose response to them is unpredictable. Rather than risk sharing a contrary opinion and being insulted, humiliated, or embarrassed, they tend to go along with the opinions expressed by other members of the group. Decisions in such groups may appear to be produced by consensus, because there is no apparent disagreement, but in fact, consensus may not be present. Because there is no group commitment and cohesion, conflict presents a threat to the group's interpersonal structure. Members try to smooth conflicts rather than resolve them. When disagreement arises, the members make quick compromises to get along. They resort to conflict-reducing techniques, such as majority rule and trade-offs. The quality of decisions made in these groups tends to be low.

The other possibility is that a great deal of verbal conflict will occur among the untrained members in a heterogeneous group, with each member insisting on his own point of view, so that the group never arrives at a decision with which everyone can be satisfied. This tends to occur most often in ad hoc groups with high-power personalities.

The variable of training in the consensus-seeking process is the most critical of all for producing synergy. In studies conducted by Dr. Jay Hall, a social scientist, trained and untrained groups were assigned the task of arriving at solutions that could be quantifiably measured; both types of groups produced synergy. In the trained groups, however, synergy occurred 75% of the time, while in the untrained groups, it occurred only 25% of the time.[8] The implications are obvious: Group leaders, facilitators, managers, supervisors, and all those who try to work with others in a participative manner need to understand the principles of training and instruct their groups in the process. A second finding was that under conditions of training, the heterogeneous groups performed better than the homogeneous groups. In fact, the broader the range of opinions presented, the better the group's chances of arriving at superior decisions. The implication here is that a group of "lemons," group members who fight and cannot agree, can be turned into "lemonade" if the facilitator trains them in the consensus-seeking process.

GUIDELINES FOR SEEKING CONSENSUS

The training required to move a group from 25% to 75% efficiency in achieving consensus is based on a set of guidelines for group behavior; it is simple and not time-consuming. The administrative dietitian who decides to use this method with his staff needs to understand, however, that it may take several weeks of regularly reminding the group of the guidelines, and interrupting each time the guidelines are not followed, before the process becomes natural to the group. These guidelines for achieving consensus in groups are as follows.

1. Everyone in the group has the responsibility and obligation to share his opinions.

2. After a group member has expressed his opinion on a particular issue, he has the right to ask others to paraphrase his comments to his satisfaction.

3. After he has been paraphrased, he may not bring up his perspective again unless he is asked to do so by another group member. Insisting on one's own point of view or blocking discussion is not allowed.

4. Everyone has the responsibility to understand the arguments and opinions of the other members, and may ask questions for clarification.

5. After all perspectives are understood, the group needs to arrive at a solution or decision with which everyone can be satisfied. In

accomplishing this task, the group may not immediately resort to the stress-reducing techniques of majority rule, trade-offs, averaging, coin-flipping, and bargaining.

6. Differences of opinion should be viewed as natural and expected. Members need to be encouraged to seek them out so that everyone is involved in the decision process. Disagreements can help the group's decision because with a wider range of information and opinions, there is a greater chance that the group will develop more adequate solutions. Frequently, when the group members suspend their own judgment, new solutions emerge that no single individual would have been able to develop alone. These solutions tend to incorporate the best points of all views—of both the majority and the minority. Such solutions tend to be synergistic. At times, however, after considerable discussion, no new solution emerges. In those instances, alternative problem-solving techniques can be applied.[8]

Alternative Problem-Solving Techniques. When a group is unable to agree on a solution, several other methods, each with its advantages and disadvantages, can be used. One method is for the leader to make the decision. The advantage is that the decision is arrived at quickly; the disadvantage is that those who dislike it may not support it. While the leader may feel that he has "won," others who feel that they have "lost" may attempt to subvert the decision or solution. Another possibility is for some members to accommodate others by no longer insisting on their preferred solution. This method will immediately relieve the group of conflict, but those who accommodated may later resent having done so and may not feel obliged to uphold the solution. Perhaps the most common method is compromise, each side giving in a little until both can agree. The problem with compromise is that often what is given up is sought back eventually. Compromise solutions tend to be short-lived. Other conflict-reducing techniques such as majority rule, trade-offs, and coin-flipping also tend to be short-lived because the members who gave up something to satisfy the immediate need for a solution feel no obligation to support the solution.

Group Participation in Decision-Making. There are both advantages and disadvantages to participative decision-making. The administrative dietitian needs to be aware of them in order to decide, on a contingency basis, when this method is appropriate.

Advantages. 1. When a manager meets with his team members one at a time, problems of communication and perceptual distortion may occur. Each time the manager discusses the issues on a one-to-one basis, his manner and language vary, with each subordinate asking questions from his own perspective. Meeting together to discuss such matters as operational activities and politics provides an opportunity for everyone to hear the same descriptions at the same time, and to ask questions, which may clarify perceptions, so that everyone shares a common understanding.

2. Interpersonal relationships and problems can be resolved, particularly when the staff is aware of the need for teamwork.

3. Motivation can be enhanced since the individuals involved in the decision may become more committed to it and may better understand how it is to be carried out. Resistance to change is lessened when individuals consider the alternative actions together and decide together on the goals and objectives for achieving change. They experience a greater commitment to changes that they themselves have either initiated or participated in developing.

4. The synergy of problem-solving can occur, allowing the group to arrive at solutions that are qualitatively superior to any that a single individual could arrive at alone.

Disadvantages. 1. Group participation in decision-making can be time consuming; however, the time spent in goal setting, problem definition, and planning can result in more rapid implementation of the solution and less resistance to change.

2. Cohesive groups can become autonomous and work against management's preferences.

3. Groups can sometimes become a way for everyone to escape the responsibility for taking action, since each person may assume that someone else is ultimately responsible.

4. The goals and interests of employees and those of management may not be compatible.

5. Employees may not be qualified to participate. Participation requires not only a desire to be involved, but also an ability to communicate insights, reactions, and desires. Not everyone possesses these skills to the same degree, and some who have the desire, but not the ability, may need to be trained.

6. Individuals whose ideas are continuously rejected can become alienated.

7. A manager may use groups as a way to manipulate employees into making the decision that he has already arrived at himself.

8. Work group involvement may raise employees' expectations that cannot always be met or that the manager did not intend, and once started, employees may want to be included in all decision-making, whether or not their participation is appropriate.

9. The hazards of "groupthink," a term explained in the next section, may emerge.

GROUPTHINK

While "synergy" refers to the phenomenon of a group being able to arrive at solutions superior to what any individual working alone could accomplish, "groupthink" refers to the phenomenon of a group stifling individual creativity to preserve the status quo. It is the mode of thinking that persons engage in when seeking concurrences becomes more important in a cohesive group than a realistic appraisal of the alternative courses of action. The symptoms of groupthink arise when group members avoid being too harsh in their judgments of their leaders' or their colleagues' ideas for the sake of preserving harmony. All members are amiable and seek complete concurrence on every important issue to avoid conflict that might spoil the cozy, group atmosphere.[9]

Dr. Irving Janis, social psychologist, is the leading expert on the groupthink phenomenon. Below are some of the remedies he suggests to prevent its occurrence. Administrative dietitians need to consider ways of adapting these practices to their own style of group facilitation with staff.[9]

1. At each meetings, the facilitator should verbalize his desire that all participants assume the role of "critical evaluator." Members need to be encouraged to look for the weaknesses in one another's arguments. The leader's acceptance of criticism from others is critical if the others are to continue the practice with him and with one another.
2. The facilitator should adopt an impartial stance instead of stating preferences and expectations at the beginning. Such a stance encourages open inquiry and impartial probing of a wide range of policy alternatives.
3. The organization should routinely set up several alternative policy planning and evaluation groups to work on the same policy question, with each group deliberating under a different leader. This practice can prevent the insulation of an ingroup.
4. Before reaching a final consensus, the group members should discuss the issues with qualified associates who are not part of the decision-making group, and should then report back to the others the results of their informal surveys.
5. The group should invite one or more outside experts to each meeting on a staggered basis and encourage the experts to challenge the views of the dominant group members.
6. At every general meeting of the group, whenever the agenda calls for an evaluation of policy alternatives, at least one member should be assigned to play the "devil's advocate," challenging the testimony of those who advocate the majority position.
7. When the group surveys policy alternatives for feasibility and effectiveness, it should from time to time divide into two or more subgroups to meet separately, under different

chairpersons, and then come back together to negotiate differences.

8. After reaching a preliminary consensus about what seems to be the best policy, the group should hold a "second-chance" meeting at which every member expresses as vividly as he can all his residual doubts. This meeting gives everyone a last opportunity to rethink the entire issue before making a definitive choice.

MEETING MANAGEMENT

This section offers the administrative dietitian several concise suggestions for exploring the "process variables" that affect staff as they work together in groups. There will be times when the administrative dietitian senses tension among his staff but is uncertain of its cause. At these times, a department meeting can be called for the specific purpose of resolving and exposing work-related problems. Knowing how to assist the group in solving problems is a responsibility of the administrative dietitian. Enlightened supervisors recognize the value in calling the group together occasionally for "process meetings."

A process meeting is one called for the specific purpose of discussing the group as a group. The items discussed include the process variables mentioned at the beginning of this chapter: how the group functions internally, how the members relate to one another, which procedures the group follows, how members communicate among themselves, and how they do their work as a group. The administrative dietitian should initiate such meetings whenever he sees a need; however, anyone in the department who sees a need for such a meeting should be encouraged to suggest it.

If the supervisor decides to call the entire group together to share his concerns about the dynamics in the work group, he should be sincere and candid in asking for their assistance, and he should schedule the meeting at an appropriate time and place. The right time is when the staff is not preoccupied with other urgent problems and when they are being paid for their time. A group should never be given too brief a time limit when the task is to discuss the dynamics of their work group.

Until the staff becomes comfortable with them, the first process meetings may be slow in starting, with people asking, "Why are we here?" After the facilitator describes his reasons for inferring tension in the group, he should remain quiet until group members begin to offer this own subjective explanations for the tension. While "process meetings" are not yet common, supervisors who do hold them regularly find that they are able to short-circuit departmental problems by giving the staff members time to vent their feelings and to resolve conflicts with one another. An underlying assumption here is that the supervisor is skilled in the conflict resolution and counseling techniques that are discussed elsewhere in this book.

A serious problem among administrators, department heads, and others who regularly need to depend on a staff for participative decision making is keeping group members motivated to participate, to follow through on assignments and tasks, and to be fully prepared prior to the meeting so that they can offer informed opinions. If there is a general problem with the group's not being prepared at meetings and the administrative dietitian is not sure what the underlying causes are, he might consider distributing a survey. The survey could be passed out prior to the meeting, with members asked to remain anonymous. The facilitator could then tabulate the results and use the data as the basis for a process meeting. Usually, the facilitator manages process meetings; however, from time to time he may wish to appoint another to moderate the meetings, especially if he observes himself talking too much or becoming defensive.

No two work groups are exactly alike or have identical problems and concerns. For that reason, facilitators should be creative in designing surveys that are tailored for their specific groups. The survey might be used to point out discrepancies between how people think the group feels about a particular work issue versus how it actually feels. The survey could also ask for opinions regarding the members' perceptions of the clarity of group goals, the degree of trust and openness within the group, the level of sensitivity and perceptiveness among group members, the amount of attention to group process, the ways in which group leadership needs are met, the ways in which decisions are made, how well the group's resources are used, and the amount of loyalty and sense of belonging in the group. As pointed out in Chapter 2, selective perception often leads individuals to infer motives and opinions that do not correspond with fact. Group discussion of survey results exposes the different perspectives existing subjectively within the group.

It may be that the group is satisfied with the status quo, and the supervisor is dissatisfied. Perhaps he objects to the fact that the staff members insist on deviating from the agenda, or that they ignore responsibilities they had agreed to at previous meetings, or that they are not prepared to discuss the issues on the agenda that had been sent to them to consider. When it is the facilitator who is dissatisfied, he should facilitate the process meeting himself, albeit very carefully. He needs to reaffirm the norms he wants, making sure that everyone understands them, and then he needs to stop people any time a norm is violated.

Even among a group of individuals who see one another regularly and do not feel any need for a formal "process meeting," there is still value in providing a time for them to relieve social concerns when they are called together for group meetings. It is a good idea for the supervisor to plan on giving them 5 to 8 minutes to settle in socially before they get down to business. Providing extra time requires that the business agenda be tailored accordingly. If 45 minutes of business have to be conducted, the facilitator needs to allow 55 minutes for the total meeting time. The group should be reminded regularly that those first minutes are intended to be social and not used as "grace time" for latecomers. Everyone is expected to arrive on time so that the social time is used for that purpose. The supervisor's arriving early to greet people provides an opportunity for individuals to inform him of any special problems or concerns.

A common inference among work groups is that the "boss" is looking for a "rubber stamp" group and is not truly interested in what the members believe. Unfortunately, the "boss" or administrator is usually the last to discover this inference. This phenomenon is called the "good news barrier to communication." An archetype common in the classic Greek tragedies of Aeschylus, Euripides, and Sophocles is that the messenger who brought the news to the king that his son had been killed in battle was then killed himself. The ancient Greek dramatists were tapping into a universal fear, which is alive and well today in the workplace. This unconscious fear causes negative situations to be described more positively to the supervisor and causes groups to fail to expose the "real" problems. It is to an administrator's advantage to be informed of the most "truthful" and objective data available. A way to foster openness in groups of staff members is to be consistently supportive, relieving the anxiety that might accompany being candid in group discussions. The staff needs to be asked for input on how the meetings could be improved. Once their suggestions are understood, as many as possible should be implemented.

Often, a common complaint among administrators regarding staff meetings is that no one seems to have anything to say. The groups seem noncreative or unwilling to generate new ideas. Suggestions on how to solve this problem might include assigning members the task of writing brief reports prior to the meeting. Including their names on the agenda next to the report topic is usually enough to inspire them to gather their thoughts beforehand. Of course, group leaders can stop the meeting at any time and dictate discussion questions to the group. After the group has been given 10 minutes to jot down some response, even in a personal shorthand, the meeting can be resumed. (Members should be reassured that no one else will read their answers.) In this way, everyone can have something to contribute. Another technique is to divide the group into small subgroups and allow each subgroup time to discuss various issues or problems. Often, individuals who are hesitant to speak up in a large group will converse with one or two others. When the large group is reconvened, the subgroup, not the hesitant individual, can give a report on its conclusions. In that way, minority opinions that might not otherwise surface may obtain recognition within the group.

At the end of a meeting, assignments for the following meetings can be distributed. The supervisor can increase the likelihood of the group following through with their assignments by asking each person to paraphrase their responsibilities for the next meeting. The act of acknowledging responsibility in the presence of the others adds pressure on the participant to complete his assigned tasks. If members do come unprepared regularly, the supervisor should consider adjourning the meeting until they are ready. Usually, this needs to be done only once for members to get the point.

Several days prior to the meeting, the facilitator should have notes sent out with the agenda to remind participants of their obligations to report, read documents, have subgroup meetings, and the like. Placing names next to agenda items acts as stimulus for members to be prepared to report at meetings.

Often, supervisors assume that they must know how to handle all problems that may occur in the work groups and at staff meetings, mistakenly believing that they are expected to have the insight, expertise, and competence to correct all problems. What they actually need to have is the humility and courage to ask for help. Supervisors need to be conscious of the various resources in their work groups and be willing to utilize the talents of group members whenever possible. Allowing individuals who may be especially competent in a particular area to share their knowledge with the others, to manage an individual group meeting, or to train subordinates involves more than just delegation. It involves showing respect for and raising the self-esteem of the individual subordinate. A supervisor must lead, but not always by leading. He can perform just as efficiently simply by seeing that the leadership takes place.

The supervisor must consider the possibility that he himself is the cause of the group members' underlying tensions or of their being unable to "gel" at meetings. Some common pitfalls among supervisors include not allowing time at the end of meetings for people to comment on how meetings might be improved, making sarcastic remarks to participants during meetings, or becoming defensive when comments about the supervisor do emerge. Group members may be unable to participate optimally and may feel frustrated with the facilitator if he neglects to do the following:

Send out agendas.
Inform the group of the core topic for the meeting.
Give assignments to individuals.

Provide essential information to participants prior to the meeting.

Inform especially resourceful individuals of how they can participate.

Provide adequate time at meetings to discuss the topic fully.

Occasionally, the supervisor finds himself in the position of selecting group members to work together on specific ad hoc organizational problems. These teams need to be selected carefully. Members need to be able to work together, and individual personalities should be a consideration. Groups should be kept as small as possible. Once these group members begin to work together, the supervisor should remain aware of their progress and of the developing group character. If and when "dead wood" becomes apparent, those members should be dropped and replaced with others who are willing to participate fully.

The reader needs to be reminded that learning to run effective meetings with staff is similar to learning to type or training for an athletic event. It requires conscientious "training" and much practice. Over time, however, the improvements are remarkable.

GROUPS AS SUPPLEMENT TO INDIVIDUAL COUNSELING

Group and individualized counseling may be used together. Even those persons who require intensive individual counseling can benefit by the examples, support, and ideas available in groups. When specialized and intense one-on-one dietary counseling does not produce the desired results, group counseling may be advantageous. When problems are mutual, the group can provide support, reinforcement, and all the advantages of synergy in solving problems. Groups also provide the resources for conducting role plays and rehearsing actions for the real world.

As used in nutritional counseling, groups differ from group therapy. Group counseling is intended to be not a form of therapy, but a format to help people find solutions to dietary problems. These solutions can then be demonstrated, attempted, and evaluated with group support.[2]

A primary goal in nutritional counseling is to promote self-sufficiency in clients. In groups where people learn basic change strategies by helping other group members design personal dietary change programs, and by encouraging mutual follow-through, this self-sufficiency goal is enhanced. Once the group understands the basic strategies, the dietitian can facilitate nondirectively, allowing the members to consult with one another.

Some consider group counseling impractical when it is limited to a single session. Behavior change requires more than one session, but a single group session may be an efficient way to give information to a group of patients or clients with similar problems. The dietitian is saved from having to explain basic concepts over and over. Being with others who share similar problems often encourages participants to change more than if they were counseled individually.

When the group is designed primarily for the dietitian to convey nutrition and dietary information, to teach principles of dietary change, and to encourage group members to use them, several principles should be incorporated into the teaching aspects of group sessions:[2]

1. The number of major points covered per meeting should be limited. The dietitian should focus all his efforts toward motivating the group to understand and use these main principles.
2. Since learning is a gradual process, teaching time in groups should be devoted to essential and necessary information. The intricate technicalities can be taught later.
3. The principles of education covered in other places in this book should be used: the goal of the session should be stated, examples should be given, and group discussion and problem solving should be stimulated. Participants should be encouraged to summarize the points learned and their intended applications of them.
4. The content should be presented and reinforced through a variety of means: written presentations, audiovisual media, role-playing, and demonstrations.
5. Group members should be required to write down or publicly verbalize short-term goals that are specific and "doable," so that they can be reviewed in the group the following week.

This chapter has stressed the necessity for dietitians to study group process and internalize the behaviors needed to participate in, facilitate, and model group interaction skills. Under proper leadership, groups can stimulate solutions and insights that individuals might not experience otherwise. Once he develops the skills needed to diagnose group needs and the ability to correct them by focusing on the group's resources, the dietitian can function as an agent of change, a communication model for the other group members, and a more effective counselor and administrator.

SUGGESTED ACTIVITIES

1. In groups of three, discuss the "best" small group experiences you have ever had. What occurred that qualifies them as superior? Describe specific behaviors of both the group's leader and the par-

ticipants that seem to have made a difference. Time should be allotted for each group to share its insights with the others.

2. In groups of three, plan to meet in three different settings over the next two days, with different seating, room size, lighting, etc. Report your observations of the effects of the environment to the entire class. Notice whether different groups had similar reactions and were influenced by the same factors. A simpler variation of this activity would be to hold a discussion for 10 minutes with the group arranged in a circle and then to continue the discussion with the group sitting in a straight row.

3. Make a list of at least three small groups in which you have been active, and describe the functions you performed in each. Compare your perceptions of yourself as a contributing group member with the perceptions that your friends or classmates had of you. Do you notice that you performed different functions in different groups? Do some functions overlap from group to group? Are your classmates in agreement with you regarding your functions within their group?

4. Thinking back to some recent experiences in group discussions, complete each of the following statements:
    A. My strengths as a group participant are . . .
    B. My strengths as a group facilitator are . . .
    C. What is keeping me from being more effective both as a participant and facilitator is . . .
    D. What I plan to improve is

5. How do you determine if needed leadership and facilitative services are being provided during a discussion? Compare your observations with those of your classmates.

6. Write a question or description of a problem, preferably from your own personal or professional experience, for which you do not have a solution. Present it to a small group and facilitate their discussion.

7. Group together 4 to 5 people who have a common problem such as needing to lose weight, needing to start eating breakfast, wanting to control excess consumption of snacks, needing to select nutritious meals, wanting to increase the fiber content of their diets, or wanting to exercise more often. State the problem, and have the group attempt to solve it.

REFERENCES

1. Brilhart, J.K.: Effective Group Discussion. 4th ed. Dubuque, IA, William C. Brown Co., 1982.

2. Rabb, C., and Tillotson, J. (eds.): Heart to Heart. Washington, DC, U.S. Dept. of Health and Human Services, 1983.
3. Mill, C.R.: Activities for Trainers: 50 Useful Designs. San Diego, University Associates, 1980.
4. Owen, A.L.: Challenges for dietitians in a high tech/high touch society. J. Am. Diet. Assoc., *84*:285, 1984.
5. Franz, M.: The dietitian: A key member of the diabetes team. J. Am. Diet. Assoc., *79*:302, 1981.
6. Baird, L.S., Schneier, C.E., and Laird, D.: Training aid for dealing with special students. *In* The Training and Development Sourcebook. Edited by L.S. Baird et al. Amherst, MA, Human Resource Development Press, 1983.
7. Beebe, S.A., and Masterson, J.T.: Communicating in Small Groups. 2nd ed. Glenview, IL, Scott, Foresman and Company, 1986.
8. Hall, J.: Decisions, decisions, decisions. Psychology Today, *5*:51, 1971.
9. Janis, I.: Groupthink. Psychology Today, *5*:43, 1971.

7

Planning Learning

Teaching is one of the major job responsibilities of all dietitians, whether they specialize in clinical, community, or administrative practice. Dietitians must be skilled in providing appropriate learning opportunities to patients, clients, and employees, to facilitate their acquisition of knowledge, attitudes, and new behaviors. Dietitians are expected to be effective teachers.

Dietitians in clinical and community practice educate clients and patients about normal nutrition, and about dietary modifications necessitated by such medical problems as cardiovascular disease and diabetes. Nutrition education has been defined as:

> ... the teaching of validated, correct nutrition knowledge in ways that promote the development and maintenance of positive attitudes toward, and actual behavioral habits of, eating nutritious foods (within budgetary and cultural constraints) that contribute to the maintenance of personal health, well-being, and productivity.[1]

The practitioner wants the individual not only to know what to do, but also to change current dietary behaviors and adopt and practice new ones. The changes sound simple: to avoid or decrease consumption of certain foods, to increase consumption of others, to change cooking methods, and the like. The internal and external forces that have shaped people's eating habits, however, are complex, are of long standing, and create barriers to successful, long-term change. Nevertheless, the final criterion of health education effectiveness has been described as "the adoption of desirable nutritional practices and their sequelae, better health and reduced disease prevalence."[2]

Many dietitians are responsible for the supervision of one or more employees. Orientation and training programs are necessary for these subordinates. An employee's on-the-job performance must meet standards acceptable to the organization, and it is the responsibility of the superior to ensure that training needs are recognized and met. The goal of training is to have the employee know his job responsibilities, and when necessary, learn and substitute new practices for current ones. The fact that an employee knows proper procedures but may not always follow them is an indication of the difficulty involved in getting a person to change.

Frequently, the terms "teaching" and "learning" are confused. Some people have the mistaken notion that if they teach something, the audience or individual learns automatically and will transfer the learning to appropriate situations. One may teach a client what the four food groups are, for example, tell him why it is important to use them in menu planning, and give him printed handouts. A passive learner who has not participated actively in the learning may not make any connection between what was taught and his own food selection or menu planning. To change behavior, education should endeavor to further the adoption of better practices. Although knowledge is a prerequisite for change, knowledge in itself does not necessarily lead to a different behavior. Motivation and intention are vital for change. A person may be knowledgeable about a healthy diet, but lack perseverance. For example, a client may be familiar with his sodium-restricted diet but may still consume salted pretzels.

Teaching factual information should not be mistaken for education. Education can be defined as the process of imparting or acquiring knowledge or skills in the context of the person's total matrix of living. Education should assist people in coping with their problems as they adapt to circumstances. The term "teaching" suggests the educator's assessment of the need for knowledge and his utilization of techniques to transfer knowledge to another individual, while the term "learning" refers to the process through which the individual acquires and stores the knowledge or skill and changes his behavior because of an interaction with, or experiences in, an educational environment. The change in behavior may be related to knowledge, attitudes, values, or skills. Health teaching and health education have been differentiated by their goals. The objective of the former, health teaching, is the "effective transmission of knowledge and skills, and that of the latter is to help people cope more effectively with problems related to their present and future health."[2]

This chapter examines theories and principles of learning and compares the characteristics of adult learners with those of children. A model or framework for planning, implementing, and evaluating learning is presented. The first three steps, which are preassessment of the learner, planning of performance objectives, and determination of the content, are examined along with information on grouping people together for learning. Discussion of additional steps in the learning process follows in Chapter 8. The question of motivation is discussed in Chapter 9.

PRINCIPLES AND THEORIES OF LEARNING

The scientific study of learning is carried on primarily by psychologists. Research has provided two major families of theories: (1) behaviorist theories, and (2) cognitive theories. Each group is discussed briefly and applied to principles of learning.

Behaviorist Theories. Behaviorist psychologists have concentrated on how individuals learn new habits or behaviors. Research has dealt with the stimulus, the response to the stimulus, and the consequences. A strengthening or weakening of behaviors as a result of the consequences has been noted. Satisfying consequences strengthen the connections between a learning stimulus and the response behavior, and increase the probability of recurrence of a behavior, while annoying states or aversive consequences weaken this connection. Thus, reinforcement and reward can be used to condition responses, but punishment is considered less effective. Behaviorists believe that to solve novel problems, learners may depend on similar stimulus-response situations, and if this does not work, they use trial and error responses.[3] The research of Pavlov, Thorndike, and Skinner is discussed more fully in Chapter 5, which the reader may wish to review.

The following are some principles of learning derived from behaviorist research:[4]

1. Arrange for the prospective learner to be successful at the activity that is to be learned, since positive consequences reinforce responses and tend to make them recur, while bad experiences decrease responses so that people avoid the learning activity. The old saying "Nothing succeeds like success" reflects this phenomenon.
2. Be sure that every time a correct response occurs, some kind of satisfier or reward follows. This reinforces the response, so that the behavior is more likely to persist.
3. If the teacher wants someone to learn something, he should wait until the person demonstrates the particular knowledge or behavior, and then reward him. Too often, incorrect responses receive attention, while correct responses are ignored. Correct actions should be reinforced.
4. Reward of a desirable response should follow immediately and not be delayed, since the strength of the connection between stimulus and response is greater with immediate reward.
5. In the early stages of learning, reinforce every desired response. Later, begin to omit some reinforcement and use an intermittent schedule of reward. When reward is overused, it loses its effect, so that after a learner has had some rewarded successes, he should be rewarded less frequently.
6. For learning sequential activities, determine the relative need for practice at each step. Some learning requires a chain of responses. Schedule the practice, including reinforcement at each step.

7. Retention depends on repetition of learning. Stimulus-response connections are strengthened with repetition.

8. Generalization of learning to similar situations suggests the importance of practice in varied contexts. If the learner is expected to respond to a variety of stimuli, practice should be given with several of the variety.

9. Knowledge of results is an effective secondary reinforcer. The learner should know his stage of progress. If he knows he is doing something properly, that knowledge reinforces the response.

10. Do not reinforce undesirable behaviors or responses. They should be ignored, which should lead to their extinction. Correct behavior should be reinforced instead.

11. Punishment is ineffective in fostering learning. It is an aversive consequence that will make the learner avoid the situation in the future.

12. Do not try to teach if the learner is tired, irritated, preoccupied, or avoiding the learning situation. The individual has to have positive conditions and be ready to learn in order to find learning satisfying.

13. Conflicts, frustrations, and barriers to learning should be recognized and resolved so that the learner is ready for a positive experience.

14. In testing the learner, the teacher should not use "trick questions" unless the learner has been familiarized with the stimulus situation. The learner should first be taught the tricks.

15. Some novel behaviors can be enhanced through imitation of models. People learn by watching the experiences of others.

Cognitive Theories. Cognitive psychologists are concerned with cognitive structures and consider "insight" a possible factor in learning to solve problems. The learner perceives a relationship, which leads to the solution of problems. Learning is discontinuous and sudden, with behavior changing when insight occurs. Cognitive learning theorists view behavior as purposive and goal-directed, rather than as a response to a stimulus, and the learner follows a sort of internal, cognitive map to a goal. The person is viewed as an active, organizing entity, rather than a passive respondent to stimuli in the environment.[3]

The following principles of learning from cognitive theory differ from behaviorist theory:

1. The learner should be active rather than passive as a listener, viewer, or responder. "Learning by doing" is emphasized.

2. Setting goals is an important motivation for learning, and successes and failures at learning determine how the learner sets future goals. Behavior is purposive.
3. Attention should be paid to careful analysis of the tasks that confront learners. The way the problem is displayed is an important condition of learning. Problems should be structured so that their features are clear to the learner.
4. The way in which knowledge is organized should be planned in advance.
5. Learning that is understood is more permanent and transferrable than rote learning.
6. Cognitive feedback must be provided to confirm correct knowledge and correct faulty learning, so that the learner is always left with the correct answer.
7. Motivation and drive are important to purposive behavior.

ADULTS AS LEARNERS

When a person accepts responsibility for teaching a client, patient, or employee, it is natural for him to think back to his own past experiences, or how he was taught in school or college. Most educational experiences were the result of pedagogy, which may be defined as the art and science of teaching children.[5,6] The teacher was an authority figure, and dependent students complied with assignments.

Adult education has challenged some of the basic ideas and approaches of pedagogy. Knowles has focused attention on beliefs about educating adults and, instead of pedagogy, uses the term "andragogy." He maintains that the basic assumptions regarding adult learners differ from those regarding child learners.[5,6] His four major assumptions for adult learners involve the following:

1. Changes in self-concept from being dependent to being self-directed.
2. The role of expanding experiences as a resource for learning.
3. Readiness to learn based on developmental tasks of social roles.
4. Orientation to learning shifting from subject matter to problem solving and from a future-oriented to a present-oriented focus.

Self-Concept. Childhood is a period of dependency. As a person matures, the self-concept changes, and the individual becomes increasingly independent and self-directed. He makes his own decisions and manages his life. Once he becomes a self-directed adult, any educational experience in which he is treated as a dependent child is a threat to his self-concept. Negative feelings may result, such as resentment or anxiety, which will interfere with learning.

Experience. As compared with a child, an adult has an increasing background of experiences, which he brings to new learning situations. This background is a resource for learning. Ignoring the adult's experience may be misinterpreted as a sign of rejection. A client who has had diabetes for 5 years, for example, has a wealth of experience that should be recognized when the dietitian discusses the diabetic diet. To ignore this prior experience and start from the beginning may annoy, bore, or possibly antagonize the client, and may place obstacles in the way of the learning process. Teaching methods such as lectures are deemphasized in adult education in favor of more participatory methods, such as discussion or projects that recognize the person's wealth of experience. Practical applications that apply learning to the individual's day-to-day life are appropriate.

Readiness. Readiness to learn differs for children and adults. Children are assumed to be ready to learn because there are subjects they ought to know about, and there are academic pressures to perform. Adults have no such pressures and are assumed to be ready to learn things required for performing their social roles in life—as spouses, employees, parents, and the like. Education of adults should be appropriate to the individual's readiness, and a timing of learning experiences needs to coincide with readiness. People are ready to learn when they are confronted by problems that they must solve. For example, a new employee may be ready to learn about his job responsibilities, but not necessarily about the history of the company. A client may not be ready to learn about his modified diet until he has accepted the fact that his medical condition and future health require it.

Orientation. A child's learning is oriented toward subjects, while an adult's learning is oriented toward solving problems. These different approaches involve different time perspectives. Because children learn about things that they will use some time in the future, the subject matter approach may be appropriate. Adults approach learning when they have a problem to solve and have an immediate need to learn. The implication is that learning should be oriented to problems or projects that the individual is currently dealing with. Adults learn what they want to learn when they want to learn it, regardless of what others want them to learn.

From an examination of various educational theories, Knowles described the appropriate conditions for learning to take place.[5,6] He suggested that the learner should feel the need to learn something, and should perceive the goals of any learning experience as his own personal goals. The adult should participate actively in planning, implementing, and evaluating learning experiences to increase his commitment to learning, and the process should make use of the person's life experiences. The physical and psychological environment needs to be comfortable. The relationship between the instructor and learner should be characterized by mutual trust, respect, and helpfulness, and the environment should encourage freedom of expression and acceptance of differences.

The professional who accepts the assumptions of "andragogy" becomes a facilitator of learning or a change agent rather than a teacher. The educator involves the learner in the process of learning and provides resources for assisting learners to acquire knowledge, information, and skills, while maintaining a supportive climate for learning.

The helping relationship was described by Tough, who investigated the self-planned learning projects of adults.[7] Tough found that when an individual initiates a learning project, he often seeks the assistance of others. As described in Tough's research, the ideal helper is warm, loving, accepting, supportive, encouraging, and friendly. He cares about the learner and his problem and takes the problem seriously. He regards the learner as an equal. In contrast to a person who wants to control, command, persuade, and influence, the ideal helper views his interaction with the learner as a dialogue with mutual interaction, listening, understanding, responding, and helping.

ENVIRONMENT

Psychological Environment. The psychological climate for learning is important, and it is determined by the approach of the educator. Openness and encouragement of questions create an informal atmosphere. A tolerance of mistakes and respect for individual and cultural differences are emphasized. Individuals should be known by their names, and respect for their opinions should be demonstrated. Collaboration and mutual assistance rather than competition should be promoted, and initial feelings of anxiety should be reduced so that they do not inhibit learning. The professional who creates this informal, supportive, and caring environment for adult learners can obtain better results than one who creates the formal, authoritative environment typical of pedagogy. If the learner has negative memories of his early experiences in school, for example, if a client or employee was ever dismissed from high school, a physical or psychological climate that reminds him of his past will create barriers to learning.

Physical Environment. One should consider not only the psychological climate, but also the physical environment. Comfort should be provided with appropriate temperature, lighting, ventilation, and comfortable chairs to create conditions that promote learning rather than inhibit it. Noise from a radio, television, telephone, or people talking may interfere with a client's or patient's attention. Individuals should be able both to see and to hear. Interaction is facilitated by seating groups of people in a circle or around a table, which allows everyone to have eye contact, as opposed to seating people in row upon row of chairs.

STEPS TO EDUCATION

Successful educational efforts that meet the needs of the adult learner include a number of interactive steps. The framework and components are:

1. Preassessment of the needs of the individual or group.
2. Planning of performance objectives that are measurable, feasible, and able to be accomplished in a stated period of time.
3. Determination of the content based on the preassessment and the objectives.
4. Selection of methods, techniques, materials, and resources appropriate to the objectives and the individual or group.
5. Implementation of the learning experiences to provide opportunities for the person to practice new information.
6. Evaluation of progress performed continuously and at stated intervals, including rediagnosis of learning needs.
7. Documentation of the results of education.

This chapter examines the first three components; Chapter 8 treats the others.

Preassessment

The first step in education is to conduct a preassessment with the client or employee. Preassessment is a diagnostic evaluation performed prior to instruction for the purpose of placement, or for establishing a starting point, and it serves to classify people regarding their current knowledge, skills, abilities, aptitudes, interests, personality, educational background, and psychological readiness to learn.

A need for learning may be defined as a gap between what the person should know and what he knows now, or the difference between how the employee should perform and his actual performance. If preassessment determines that an individual already has some knowledge, as in the case of a client with long-term diabetes who knows the exchange system, more advanced material is indicated. One determines in advance how much the individual already knows, since it would be a waste of everyone's time to repeat known information, which could lead to boredom or lack of attention on the part of the learner. Does the client have the intellectual capabilities to receive the instruction? Some people are unable to read, and such limitations require that the instruction be planned at the client's level. Educational planning should be based on the dietitian's preassessment of the client's or employee's knowledge and ability.

Psychological preassessment is also necessary since the dietitian must understand the attitudes that influence the client's or employee's behavior. Attitudes are thought to be predispositions for action. Problems in learning may not be cognitive, or caused by deficits in knowledge; the cause and cure may be found in the affective domain, or in attitudes, values, and beliefs. Nutrition behaviors are the result of many motivations, and having nutrition information does not necessarily mean that the information will be applied.[1] For example, the hospitalized patient who has just learned of his diagnosis of chronic illness is unlikely to learn much about a prescribed dietary treatment at that moment. He may be thinking: "Why me?" "What did I do to deserve this?" "How will this affect my job? my lifestyle? my marriage?" A new employee may feel high levels of anxiety, which may interfere with learning for the first few days on the job. Anxiety may arise whenever a superior trains a subordinate. "What does the superior think about me?" "He will think I am dumb if I don't understand, so I had better pretend I do understand." These feelings are barriers to learning that must be reduced or eliminated prior to teaching.

In some situations, preassessment may be handled by interviewing. One may inquire: "Have you been on a diet before?" "Can you tell me what foods are good sources of potassium?" "Can you explain the relationship between your diet and your health?" In general, the line of questioning should be based on what the person needs to know. Interviewing may be used with employees as well. "Have you ever used a meat slicer before?" "Can you show me how you set tables at the restaurant where you worked previously?"

In more formal situations, a preassessment test may be developed and administered. The purpose of the test is to evaluate the individual's capabilities before instruction begins and to identify what the individual already knows. Pretest results may be compared later with posttest results, after instruction has been completed. Preassessment is most necessary when the dietitian is unfamiliar with the knowledge, ability, and values of the client, patient, or employee.

In business, training and development programs are planned to meet present and future goals and objectives. Training provides specific skills, often motor or manual in nature, under the guidance of established personnel so that employees meet standards acceptable to the organization. Training is needed by new employees and by current employees accepting new assignments, such as after promotion or transfer. A need for training may be described as the difference between actual and desired performance. Training needs may be determined in a number of ways, for example, by discussing problems with subordinates; by directly observing the work; by asking questions of employees; by seeing what is done correctly and especially what is not; by examining reports of accidents, incidents, grievances, turnover, productivity, and quality control and assurance; and by administering attitude surveys.[8-10] One may ask, "What are the attitudes, skills, and knowledge employees need to perform their jobs effectively?"

Performance Objectives

Developing precise statements of goals can help to organize one's thinking regarding the purpose of the instruction, i.e., what is to be learned. One needs to decide what is to be learned prior to selecting the methods and techniques to accomplish it. References to goal statements are found in the literature under the terms "behavioral objectives," "performance objectives," and "measurable objectives." Because the term "behavioral objectives" may be erroneously confused with behaviorism, the term "performance objectives" is used in this chapter. Written performance objectives are helpful tools in planning, implementing, and evaluating learning.

A well-stated performance objective communicates the teacher's instructional intent for the learner. It specifies the learner's behavior after instruction is completed. Writing performance objectives has many advantages. It results in less ambiguity regarding what is to be learned. Also, clear performance objectives make it possible to assess the degree to which the objectives have been achieved. Both the teacher and the learner benefit from clearer instructions. When the learner knows what he is supposed to learn, it does not come as a surprise. Learners should not be kept guessing about what should be learned or about what is important. This would be a waste of their time.

Thus, initial effort is devoted to delineating the intended results of instruction for the learner, rather than to determining the methods or processes of learning. One first defines the ends and then explores the means to the ends. Instruction must benefit the learner, not the teacher, so one must focus initially on the results in the learner. If clear objectives are not written, the instructor cannot select content or materials for instruction. One cannot select an educational filmstrip, for example, without knowing what it is to accomplish. As pointed out by Mager, "If you're not sure where you're going, you're liable to end up someplace else."[11]

Objectives should focus on the person learning. The following objective is poorly stated: "The dietitian will teach the client his diet." Note that this statement focuses on what the instructor will do, and not on what the client or learner will do. The following is preferred because it focuses on the client: "The client will be able to plan appropriate menus using his sodium-restricted diet."

One of the most useful guides to writing performance objectives was published by Mager.[11] A key to writing measurable performance objectives is the selection of verbs that describe the desired outcome. Some verbs are vague and subject to misinterpretation, as in the following objectives:

To know (is able to know which foods contain potassium)
To understand (is able to understand that foods high in potassium should be consumed daily when certain medications are prescribed)
To appreciate (is able to appreciate the importance of following the dietitian's instructions)

In the written objective for "to know," it is not clear whether "knowing" means that the client will purchase foods high in potassium, consume foods high in potassium, be able to relate which foods are high in potassium, or recognize them on a list. "Understanding" could mean being able to recall reasons, being able to read an article about it, or being able to apply knowledge to one's own situation. The meanings of knowing, understanding, and appreciating are not clear.

Instead, one should select verbs that describe what the person is able to do after learning has taken place. Note that the phrase "is able to" is used, and that "the learner" is understood to precede this phrase, since one is describing what the person will be capable of doing. Another method involves starting with an action verb. The first two examples are rewritten from the unsatisfactory objectives in the previous list. Better verbs to use include the following:

To recall (is able to recite five good food sources of potassium)
To explain (is able to explain why foods high in potassium should be consumed)
To write (is able to list the four food groups)
To compare (is able to compare the nutrient needs of an adult woman with those of a pregnant woman)
To identify (is able to identify on the menu those foods that are permitted)
To solve or *use* (is able to plan menus using a diet instruction sheet)
To demonstrate (is able to demonstrate the use of the mixer)
To operate (is able to slice meat on the meat slicer)

Mager noted that three characteristics improve written objectives: (1) performance, (2) conditions, and (3) criterion.[11] The performance is what the learner will be able to do after instruction has been given. The second characteristic describes under what conditions the performance is to occur. Finally, a criterion tells how good the learner's performance must be to be acceptable. Conditions and criterion may not be included in all objectives. In general, the more that can be specified, the better the objective and the more likely that the patient, client, or employee will learn what the dietitian intends.

Performance. The performance component of an objective describes the activity in which the learner will be engaged. The performance may be visible or heard, such as listing, reciting, explaining, or operating equipment, or invisible, such as identifying or solving a problem. While overt or visible performance may be seen or heard directly, invisible or covert performance requires that the learner be asked to say or do something visible to determine whether or not the objective is satisfied and learning has taken place. In invisible performance, one adds an indicator behavior to the objective, for example:

Is able to identify the parts of the meat slicer (on a diagram or
    verbally)

Identifying is invisible until the learner is asked to identify the parts on a diagram or to recite them verbally, which is the indicator behavior. The major intent or performance should be stated using an active verb, and an indicator should be added if the performance cannot be seen or heard.

Conditions. Once the performance has been clearly stated, one may ask whether or not there are specific circumstances or conditions under which the performance will be observed. The conditions describe the setting, equipment, or cues associated with the behavior. With what resources will the learner be provided? What will be withheld? Conditions are in parentheses in the following examples:

(Given the disassembled parts of a meat slicer) is able to reassemble the parts in correct sequence.

(Using the diabetic diet menu for tomorrow) is able to select the proper foods in the correct quantities.

(Given a list of foods including both good and poor sources of potassium), is able to identify the good sources.

(Given a copy of a sodium-restricted diet) is able to plan a menu for a complete day.

(Without looking at the diet instruction form) is able to describe an appropriate dinner menu.

(Without the assistance of the dietitian) is able to explain the foods a pregnant woman should eat on a daily basis.

These objectives give a more accurate and complete picture of the exact performance expected of a learner. While every objective may not have conditions, it should include enough information to make clear exactly what performance is expected.

Criterion. Once the end performance has been described and the conditions, if any, under which it will be observed have been described, a criterion may or may not be added. The criterion describes a level of achievement, that is, how well the learner should be able to perform. It is a standard with which to measure performance. Possible standards include speed, accuracy, quality, and percentage of correct answers.[11]

A time limit can be used to describe the speed criterion. This is necessary only when speed is important, and if it is, it should be included in the objective. The following are examples:

Is able to type (50 words per minute).
Is able to reassemble the meat slicer (in 5 minutes or less).
Is able to complete a diet history (in 20 minutes).

For objectives that require the development of skill over a period of time, one must determine how much time is reasonable in the initial learning period as opposed to the time needed when the skill is well developed. A new employee cannot be expected to perform a task as rapidly as an experienced person.

While speed is one type of standard, a second is accuracy. Accuracy should communicate how well the learner needs to perform for his performance to be considered competent. Examples include:

Is able to type 50 words per minute (with five errors or less).
Is able to identify good sources of potassium (with 80% accuracy), given a list of foods including both good and poor sources of potassium.
Is able to plan a menu for a complete day (with no errors), given a copy of a sodium-restricted diet.
Is able to calculate the carbohydrate in the diabetic diet (within 5 grams).

If the learner is expected to perform with a degree of accuracy, this criterion should be included in the objective.

After considering whether speed and accuracy are important, one should examine the quality of the performance to assess what constitutes an acceptable performance. It is easier to communicate quality when objective standards are available to both the learner and the instructor. Any acceptable deviation from the standards can then be determined. Examples of such standards are as follows.

Is able to reassemble the meat slicer (according to the steps
in the task analysis).

Is able to measure the amount of sanitizer (according to the
directions on the label).

Is able to substitute foods on a diabetic menu (using the diabetic exchanges).

In these examples, the quality of performance has been stated according to a known standard.

Domains of Learning. After developing skill in writing measurable
performance objectives, one should consider the range of objectives
that may be written. Objectives have been organized by taxonomies
or classification systems to focus on precision in writing, and one
may examine the range of possible outcomes desired from instruction. There are three taxonomies: (1) the cognitive domain, (2) the
affective domain, and (3) the psychomotor domain.

Cognitive Domain. A taxonomy of educational objectives in the
cognitive domain was published by Bloom and others.[12] The cognitive domain involves the acquisition and utilization of knowledge
or information and the development of intellectual skills and abilities.
According to Bloom and co-authors, the cognitive domain has six
major levels or categories and a number of subcategories as shown
in the following: [12]

1.0 KNOWLEDGE
    1.10 Knowledge of specifics
    1.20 Knowledge of ways and means of dealing with specifics
    1.30 Knowledge of the universals and abstractions in a field

2.0 COMPREHENSION
    2.10 Translation
    2.20 Interpretation
    2.30 Extrapolation

3.0 APPLICATION

4.0 ANALYSIS
    4.10 Analysis of elements
    4.20 Analysis of relationships
    4.30 Analysis of organizational principles

5.0 SYNTHESIS
    5.10 Production of a unique communication
    5.20 Production of a plan, or proposed set of operations
    5.30 Derivation of a set of abstract relations

6.0 EVALUATION
   6.10 Judgments in terms of internal evidence
   6.20 Judgments in terms of external criteria

The classes are arranged from simple to complex, from concrete to more abstract, and the objectives in any one class are likely to be built on the behaviors in the previous class. The subcategories help to define the major headings further and make them more specific.

The educational planner needs to think beyond the simplest and most abstract levels of knowledge and comprehension and to write objectives at the higher, more concrete levels. Without examining the possibility of writing higher-level objectives, one may tend to think only in terms of knowledge and comprehension, which are the easiest objectives to write. The learner may then be denied the opportunity of applying knowledge or of using it in solving problems and will be reduced to memorizing facts. In nutrition education, for example, knowing facts is necessary, but the client also needs the ability to analyze food labels, to synthesize all information learned so that he may tell others about it, and to evaluate nutritional information in making wise food choices. In the following discussion of the six levels in the taxonomy, examples of objectives are given.

KNOWLEDGE. At the lowest level in the cognitive domain, knowledge involves the remembering and recall of information. This includes the recall of specific bits of information, terminology, and facts, such as dates, events, and places, chronological sequences, methods of inquiry, trends over time, processes, classification systems, criteria, principles, and theories.

Example: Is able to list foods high in sodium.

COMPREHENSION. The second level, comprehension, is the lowest level of understanding. It involves knowing what is communicated by another person and being able to use the information communicated. The use of information may include translation, restatement or paraphrase, interpretation, summarization or rearrangement of the information, and extrapolation or extension of the given information to determine implications or consequences.

Example: Is able to explain (verbally or in writing) why certain foods are excluded on the diabetic diet.

APPLICATION. At the level of application, one is able to use information, principles, or ideas in concrete situations. Knowledge is understood sufficiently to be able to apply it.

Example: Is able to plan a sodium-restricted menu for the day.

ANALYSIS. This level entails the breakdown of information into its parts to identify the elements, the interaction between elements, and the organizing principles or structure. Relationships may be made among ideas.

Example: Is able to analyze the nutrition labeling on a food product.

SYNTHESIS. Synthesis requires the re-assembling of elements or parts to form a new whole. One may assemble a unique verbal or written communication, a plan of operation, or a set of abstract relations to explain data.

Example: Is able to explain the low-cholesterol diet accurately to a friend.

EVALUATION. At the highest level in the cognitive taxonomy, evaluation is the ability to judge the value of material. Such judgment requires the use of criteria, which may be internal criteria, such as logical accuracy or consistency, or external criteria, such as external standards.

Example: Is able to evaluate a nutrition article from the daily newspaper.

Affective Domain. The affective domain deals with changes in attitudes, values, beliefs, appreciation, and interests. Often, one wants a client or employee not only to comprehend what to do, but also to value it, accept it, and find it important. Attitudes and beliefs about food are widely recognized as important determinants of an individual's food habits. According to Johnson and Johnson, the purpose of nutrition education is "to create informed consumers who value good nutrition and consume nutritious foods throughout their lives."[1] When imparting information fails to bring about behavior change, the common response is to redouble efforts to teach facts and explain why something should be done. Instead, the examination of attitudes and values should be considered.

The affective domain involves a process of internalization. It categorizes the inner growth that occurs as people become aware of, and later adopt, the attitudes and principles that assist in forming the value judgments that guide conduct. For the client learning about prenatal nutrition, the instructor may desire the person not only to be knowledgeable (cognitive domain) about the proper foods to eat during pregnancy, but also to value that the knowledge so much (affective domain) that she eats nutritious foods and practices good nutrition. An objective in one domain may have a component in another. Cognitive objectives may have an affective component, and affective objectives may have a cognitive one.

Affective objectives are more nebulous and resist precise definition; therefore, evaluation of their achievement is more difficult. The educational planner may find it a formidable task to describe affective behaviors involving internal feelings and emotions, but they are as important as overt behaviors. Because affective behaviors are more difficult to express, most written objectives express cognitive behaviors.

Krathwohl and others published a taxonomy of educational objectives in the affective domain.[13] It includes five categories and a number of subcategories:

1.0 RECEIVING (ATTENDING)
    1.1 Awareness
    1.2 Willingness to receive
    1.3 Controlled or selected attention

2.0 RESPONDING
    2.1 Acquiescence in responding
    2.2 Willingness to respond
    2.3 Satisfaction in response

3.0 VALUING
    3.1 Acceptance of a value
    3.2 Preference for a value
    3.3 Commitment

4.0 ORGANIZATION
    4.1 Conceptualization of a value
    4.2 Organization of a value system

5.0 CHARACTERIZATION BY A VALUE OR VALUE COMPLEX
    5.1 Generalized set
    5.2 Characterization

The ordering of classes describes a process by which a value progresses from a level of mere awareness or perception to levels of greater complexity until it becomes an internal part of one's outlook on life, which guides or controls behavior. This internalization may occur in varying degrees, and may involve conformity or nonconformity. At higher levels, behavior may be so ingrained that it is an unconscious rather than a conscious response, and responses may be produced consistently in the absence of external authorities, and in spite of barriers. Thus, a client may eventually select a proper diet without thinking about it at the conscious level.

RECEIVING. At the lowest level of the affective domain, the learner is willing to receive certain phenomena or stimuli. Receiving represents a willingness to attend to what the teacher is presenting. The learner may move from a passive level of awareness or consciousness, to a neutral willingness to tolerate the situation rather than to avoid it, and then to an active level of controlled or selected attention despite distractions.

Example: Is able to listen to instructions on diabetic diets.

RESPONDING. The second level, responding, indicates a desire on the part of the learner to become involved in, or committed to, a subject or activity. At the lowest level of responding, the learner may passively acquiesce, or at least comply, in response to the teacher. At a higher level, a willingness to respond or voluntarily make a commitment to his chosen response is evident. Finally, a feeling of satisfaction or pleasure in response involves an internalization on the part of the learner.

Example: Is able to read diet materials with interest and ask questions.

VALUING. At the third level, valuing, the learner believes that the information or behavior has worth, and he values it based on his personal method of assessment. When the value has been slowly internalized or accepted, the learner displays a behavior consistent with the value. When something is valued, motivation is not based on external authorities or the desire to obey, but on an internal commitment. The learner may demonstrate acceptance of a value, preference for a value, or commitment and conviction.

Example: Is able to select a nutritious meal from the cafeteria line.

ORGANIZATION. At this level, the learner discovers situations in which more than one value is appropriate. Individual values are incorporated into a total network of values, and at the level of conceptualization, a learner relates new values to those he already holds. New values must be organized into an ordered relationship with the current value system. Perhaps a client has valued eating whatever he wants, for example. If the dietitian is teaching a client a new diet, he has to learn a new value (different foods) and change an old one (some of his current eating patterns).

Example: Is able to discuss plans for following a new diet.

CHARACTERIZATION. The highest level, characterization, indicates that the values have been internalized for a sufficient time to control behavior, and the individual acts consistently over time. A generalized set is a predisposition to act or perceive events in a certain way. At the highest level of internalization, beliefs or ideas are integrated with internal consistency.

Example: Is able to select only those foods permitted on the diet at all times.

Behavioral change in the affective domain takes place gradually over a period of time, whereas cognitive change may occur more rapidly. Affective change may take days, weeks, or months at the higher levels.

Psychomotor Domain. The psychomotor domain involves the development of motor or manual skills. Knowledge and attitudes may be necessary to perform these skills. For example, one could not drive a car or operate a meat slicer, tasks requiring manual skills, without some basic knowledge of the equipment. The authors that developed the cognitive and affective domains did not develop a taxonomy for the psychomotor domain, but more than one such system has been published.[14,15] The performance of motor action proceeds to increasingly complex steps. Simpson's seven levels and subcategories are as follows:[14]

1.00 PERCEPTION
    1.10 Sensory stimulation
        1.11 Auditory
        1.12 Visual
        1.13 Tactile
        1.14 Taste
        1.15 Smell
        1.16 Kinesthetic
    1.20 Cue Selection
    1.30 Translation

2.00 SET
    2.10 Mental set
    2.20 Physical set
    2.30 Emotional set

3.00 GUIDED RESPONSE
    3.10 Imitation
    3.20 Trial and error

4.00 MECHANISM

5.00 COMPLEX OVERT RESPONSE
    5.10 Resolution of uncertainty
    5.20 Automatic performance

6.00 ADAPTATION

7.00 ORIGINATION

PERCEPTION. The lowest level of the psychomotor domain is perception. It involves becoming aware of objects by means of the senses—hearing, seeing, touching, tasting, and smelling—and by muscle sensations or activation. The learner must select which cues to respond to in order to perform a task. He then must mentally translate these selected cues into action.

Example: Is able to recognize a need to learn how to use the meat slicer.

SET. The second level, set, suggests a readiness for performing a task. In addition to being ready mentally, the learner must be ready physically, by positioning the body, and emotionally, by having a favorable attitude or willingness to learn the task.

Example: Is able to demonstrate readiness to learn to use the meat slicer.

GUIDED RESPONSE. The third level is guided response. The teacher guides the learner during the activity, emphasizing the individual components of a more complex skill. The subcategories include imitation of the teacher and trial and error until the task can be performed accurately. Performance at this level may initially be crude and imperfect.

Example: Is able to practice the steps in using the meat slicer under supervision.

MECHANISM. Mechanism, the fourth level, refers to habitual response. At this stage of learning, the learner demonstrates an initial degree of proficiency in performing the task, which results from some practice.

Example: Is able to use the meat slicer properly.

COMPLEX OVERT RESPONSE. The fifth level of complex overt response suggests that a level of skill has been attained over time in performing the task. Work is performed smoothly and efficiently without error. Two subcategories are resolution of uncertainty, in which a task is performed without hesitation, and automatic performance. Performance is characterized by accuracy, control, and speed.

Example: Is able to demonstrate skill in using the meat slicer.

ADAPTATION/ORIGINATION. Adaptation requires altering motor activity in new but similar situations, such as in adapting slicing procedures to a variety of different foods on the meat slicer. The final level, origination, refers to the creation of new physical acts.

In understanding the psychomotor domain, it may be helpful to recall the process of learning to drive an automobile, responding to physical and visual stimulation, feeling mentally and emotionally ready to drive, learning parallel parking by trial and error under the guidance of an instructor, developing a degree of skill, and finally starting the car and driving without having to think of the steps. With time, sufficient skill is developed so that the person can adapt quickly in new situations on the road and create new responses automatically.

Using the taxonomies ensures that the objectives of learning are not limited to the lowest levels, that is, to the recall of facts or to the cognitive domain only. The taxonomies assist the educational planner in thinking of higher levels of knowledge, which may be more appropriate behaviors for the learner. They also serve to remind the planner that there are interrelationships among the three domains. The dietitian should be concerned not only that the client can plan menus using his diet, but also that he thinks that the diet is important enough to his health to follow it. An employee needs not only to know sanitation procedures, but also to value them.

Adoption of Innovations

The Cooperative Extension Service of the U.S. Department of Agriculture and other groups have used a model to promote the adoption of innovations.[16] The process by which adults adopt new ideas and practices involves five stages:

1. *Awareness.* A person becomes aware of a new idea, practice, or procedure. Note that this is the same as level 1.1 in the affective domain.
2. *Interest.* A person is concerned enough to seek further information about something, is aware of his current behavior, and is willing to discuss it. He sees possibilities for the use of something new.
3. *Evaluation.* A person mentally weighs the advantages and disadvantages of the new idea. He asks, "Can I do it?"
4. *Trial.* A person tries or tests the usefulness of the new idea or practice on a small scale once or twice. It is still a low priority.
5. *Adoption (or rejection).* A person performs the innovative behavior consistently as a habitual procedure, indicating that it is accepted, highly valued, and found to be satisfying.

Nutrition education and employee education are incomplete until stage five is reached. People learn only what they want to learn, and adopt innovative behaviors to satisfy the basic needs for survival, or to achieve some personal goal. Innovations are more readily adopted if they offer sufficient advantage over current practices, if they are compatible with current practices, if they are easy to understand and to use, if they can be divided into smaller units for trial, and if their benefits are clearly and quickly demonstrated. Nutrition education rates poorly according to some of these criteria.[17] Research findings suggest that reaching the level of adoption requires considerable communication and a lengthy time span. It may be unrealistic to expect new behaviors to be adopted from short-term educational endeavors. A compromise dietary regimen or the achievement of one or two goals for change may not be what the professional considers best, but limited benefits may be preferable to risking total abandonment of a dietary regimen.[2]

Determining Content

A close examination of the objectives can help to identify the content of the instruction. The objective states what the learner will be able to do when instruction is complete and directs attention to the appropriate content. The preassessment may have eliminated certain objectives as unnecessary, and those that remain should be examined in planning content. Some learners may need to start at the lowest level in the taxonomy, while those who have already mastered the lower-level objectives are ready for those at higher levels.

Organizing Training Groups

Learning may take place individually or in groups. Groups are advantageous in that they save time and provide opportunities for people to share experiences. Those who are successful in making dietary changes can model behaviors and discuss information with those who have been unsuccessful. The more complex the information to be learned, the greater the need to discuss it in groups.

Even when one individual is involved, the dietitian should consider whether others should be present. In nutrition counseling and education, the individual responsible for purchasing the food and preparing the meals should be present. When a child is placed on a modified diet, such as a diabetic diet, usually the mother requires instruction as well, since her cooperation is essential to the child's successful adherence to the diet.

Training sessions for employees may be organized in several ways. Frequently, all new employees are grouped together for initial orientation and training. Although current employees may be grouped by age, educational level, amount of experience, or job title, the best grouping probably occurs when employees with similar learning needs are trained together. Waitresses may require sessions on sanitary dish and utensil handling, for example, while cooks may need classes on sanitary food handling. The learning needs of employees differ according to their job content and level of current knowledge. The preassessment should show differences in knowledge levels and should assist in making grouping decisions.

Another question is whether supervisors should be grouped in the same classes as their employees. One disadvantage of such a grouping is that the employees may be reluctant to participate by asking questions when the superior is present. The final decision rests on the size of the group. There is more opportunity for individual participation in groups of 10 to 15 than in groups of 30 to 50 or more.

This chapter has explored the initial steps in planning learning. After preassessment has been completed, performance objectives should be written in the cognitive, affective, and psychomotor domains. Either individual or group instruction may be organized. The content of instruction may be determined from an examination of the objectives. Chapter 8 explores the remaining steps in the framework for education.

SUGGESTED ACTIVITIES

1. Make a list of questions you would ask in the preassessment of knowledge on some subject with which you are familiar.

2. Write three performance objectives using active verbs to describe behavior.

3. Write examples of performance objectives containing conditions and a criterion.

4. Write examples of objectives in various levels of the cognitive, affective, and psychomotor domains. Note overlap from one domain to another.

5. Decide which of the following performance objectives are well-written.
   A. Presented with a menu, the patient will be able to circle appropriate food selections according to his diet.
   B. At the close of the series of classes, the clients will be more positively disposed toward following their diets.
   C. After counseling, the patient will know which foods he should eat and which he should not.
   D. The patient will be able to explain the diebetic diet to her husband.

6. Examine the following objectives and decide whether each cocerns primarily the cognitive, affective, or psychomotor domains.
   A. All clerical staff will be able to type 50 words per minute without errors.
   B. Given a series of objectives, the student will be able to classify them according to the taxonomies in the chapter.
   C. At the end of the session, clients will request more weight control classes.

Answers appear on the following page.

Answers:

5. A and D.
6A. Psychomotor.
6B. Cognitive.
6C. Affective

REFERENCES

1. Johnson, D.W., and Johnson, R.T.: Nutrition education: A model for effectiveness, a synthesis of research. J. Nutr. Ed., *17*:S1, 1985.
2. Hochbaum, G.M.: Behavior and education. *In* Nutrition, Lipids, and Coronary Heart Disease. Edited by R. Levy et al. New York, Raven Press, 1979.
3. Swenson, L.: Theories of Learning. Belmont, CA, Wadsworth Publ. Co., 1980.
4. Bugelski, B.: The Psychology of Learning Applied to Teaching. 2nd ed. Indianapolis, Bobbs-Merrill, 1971.
5. Knowles, M.S.: The Adult Learner: A Neglected Species. 2nd ed. Houston, Gulf Publ. Co., 1978.
6. Knowles, M.S.: The Modern Practice of Adult Education. New York, Association Press, 1970.
7. Tough, A.: The Adult's Learning Projects. Toronto, The Ontario Institute for Studies in Education, 1971.
8. Laird, D.: Approaches to Training and Development. Reading, MA, Addison-Wesley, 1978.
9. Morrison, J.: Determining training needs. *In* Training and Development Handbook. 2nd ed. Edited by R. Craig. New York, McGraw-Hill, 1976.
10. Rose, J.C.: Handbook for Health Care Food Service Management. Rockville, MD, Aspen Publ., 1984.
11. Mager, R.F.: Preparing Instructional Objectives. 2nd ed. Belmont, CA, Fearon Publ., 1975.
12. Bloom, B.S., Engelhart, M., Furst, E., et al. Taxonomy of Educational Objectives. Handbook I: Cognitive Domain. New York, David McKay, 1956.
13. Krathwohl, D., Bloom, B.S., and Masia, B.: Taxonomy of Educational Objectives. Handbook II: Affective Domain. New York, David McKay, 1964.
14. Simpson, E.: The classification of educational objectives in the psychomotor domain. Illinois Teacher of Home Econ., *10*:110, 1966.
15. Harrow, A.: A Taxonomy of the Psychomotor Domain. New York, David McKay, 1972.
16. Nestor, J., and Glotzer, J.: Teaching Nutrition. Cambridge, MA, Abt Books, 1981.
17. Yarbrough, P.: Communication theory and nutrition education research. J. Nutr. Ed., *13*:S16, 1981.

8

Implementing and Evaluating Learning

The initial steps in planning learning, discussed in Chapter 7, include a preassessment of the learner's current knowledge and competencies, the development of performance objectives in the cognitive, affective, and psychomotor domains, and the determination of the content to be learned. This chapter discusses the selection and implementation of appropriate learning activities for the cognitive, affective, and psychomotor domains. The sequence of material is also considered. In addition, plans for the evaluation of the results of learning and for documentation are also discussed, as these steps are necessary to complete the educational process.

SELECTING AND IMPLEMENTING LEARNING ACTIVITIES

Various methods and techniques of educational presentation are available to assist adults in reaching the objectives of learning. Techniques are defined as "the ways in which the educator facilitates learning."[1] They establish a relationship between the teacher and the learner, and between the learner and what he is learning. They include lectures, discussions, simulation, demonstrations, and the like. All are not equally effective in facilitating learning, and each has its advantages and disadvantages, its uses and limitations. In deciding which technique is appropriate, the educator may be guided by several factors. These include availability, cost, and one's previous experience or degree of success with the technique. In addition, an examination of the performance objectives may suggest which approach is most appropriate, as methods and techniques may differ for the cognitive, affective, and psychomotor domains. Learner preference should also be considered. All factors being equal, one should select the technique that requires the most active participation of the learner. As Confucius said:

> I hear and I forget,
> I see and I remember,
> I do and I understand.

Lecture. The lecture is the presentation technique most familiar to people. It has been used for years as a method of transferring knowledge—the lowest level in the cognitive domain—from the teacher to the learner, especially in situations where there are large numbers of learners and a great deal of information to be communicated. In spite of the advantages of efficiency, a major drawback to lectures is that there is no guarantee that the material is learned and remembered since the learner is a passive participant whose learning depends on listening. This may be the least effective technique. While many educated people may respond positively to lectures because of long experience with this mode, people with less education may learn better with other methods. Their attention may wane quickly, especially if the lecture is dull, and new information may be rapidly forgotten. Furthermore, lectures do not meet the requirements of adult education, or "andragogy," for self-directed learning and problem-solving approaches (see Chapter 7, "Adults as Learners"). When lectures are employed, ample time should be given for a question-and-answer or discussion period.

Discussion. In discussion techniques, whether on a one-to-one basis or in groups, the learner is an active participant, and he internalizes the knowledge through his responses. Discussion may be guided by the dietitian's raising open-ended questions or key issues, or it may be more group-centered if individuals are fairly well acquainted.[2] Debates and panel discussions, in which several people with specific knowledge informally discuss or debate an assigned topic in front of a larger group, are other approaches. The basis for discussion may be common experiences, problems, or topics that were preannounced so that the group has prepared, or case studies of real-life situations, which are developed. For best results, seating should be arranged in a circle so that everyone can see and hear one another, and so that the teacher can participate as a member of the group. There is more opportunity for participation in smaller group sizes of 10 to 15, since increased size means less opportunity for participants to speak and influence others.[2] While it is more time-consuming than lecture, discussion may be more interesting for learners, and thus more motivating, especially with higher-level cognitive objectives and with affective objectives. Discussion and oral summarization facilitate and promote the individual's acquisition and retention of information. When people study alone, or are passive listeners, some cognitive processing may not take place.

Simulation. Simulation of real situations may also be considered, and several means of representation may be utilized, such as scenarios, in-basket exercises, critical incidents, and role-playing. Simulation may be based on scenarios or models of real-life problems. In-basket exercises test the learner's ability to handle day-to-day challenges. The technique has been used to simulate a supervisor's decision-making ability in handling problems that are placed in the in-basket on his desk each day. Written memos, notes, requests, or reports are given to an individual and require him to make decisions. Critical incidents also require the learner's responses to specific situations. Emergencies or unusual incidents are used, and the learner has to provide a response in handling the situation. The use of role-playing, in which two or more persons dramatize assigned parts or roles simulating real-life situations, is another possibility. This is followed by discussion of the problem, ideas, feelings, and emotional reactions, as for example, role-playing of an employee disciplinary problem. While time-consuming, simulations may be helpful in providing opportunities for learners to make a connection between theory and practice, to engage in critical thinking, and to develop problem-solving and coping skills. Simulation may be used with both cognitive and affective objectives.[3]

Demonstration. A demonstration may be used to show how something is done, or to explore processes, ideas, or attitudes.[2] Usually, the learner observes as the instructor makes the presentation. The demonstration may be a dramatic learning experience if the learner's attention is held and may be appropriate for any type of learning objective. If skills are demonstrated, the learner will need an opportunity to try the skill at a later time. Sometimes, duplicate work operations are set up independently of the work site and are used for training.

Audio-Visual Aids. An effective media presentation can enhance learning by providing variety and improving memory through visual stimulation. One may include the use of audio-visual aids, such as videotape and television, slides, films, flip charts, posters, chalk board, overhead transparencies, food models, and audiotapes. The appropriateness of such material to the learning situation, and to the individual or group, should be considered. A videotape of one's own setting, for example, would probably foster better learning among employees than one that is purchased. Other teacher-made materials, such as charts, exhibits, and handouts may be effective aids. Such materials are an adjunct to learning and should not be considered the total learning experience.

Other techniques to promote learning include programmed instruction, computer instruction, laboratory experiences, apprenticeship, job rotation, job enlargement, and personal reading.

Techniques for Different Domains. For learning in the cognitive domain, most of the foregoing techniques may be effective. There are additional factors to consider in fostering learning in the affective and psychomotor domains.

In the affective domain, the educator seeks to influence the learner's interests, attitudes, and values. This cannot be accomplished in an hour or a day, but requires ongoing contact. At the lowest level in the affective domain, receiving and awareness, the professional may gain the learner's attention through the use of audio-visual materials or guided discussion. At higher levels where the adoption of new attitudes and values is important, the learner must participate more fully. Attitudes are acquired through interpersonal influences, and commitments that are made public are more likely to be adopted than those that are private.[4] Discussion in a group or where experiences are shared, discussion of case studies or critical incidents, and role-playing may be effective, especially if they lead to high self-awareness and public commitment, and if people perceive that all members of the group support new attitudes and behaviors. Active oral summarization following discussion is recommended because it leads to more elaborate thinking and integration into the person's conceptual framework.

Effective instructional strategies to influence deeper-level learning of nutrition leading to modification of attitudes and dietary behaviors have been recommended. Strategies promoting the active involvement of participants and interpersonal interaction in a group, which are related to the social context, help to achieve deeper-level learning, attitude modification, and behavioral change. The strategies suggested to accomplish this include (1) cooperative learning, (2) inquiry learning, (3) nutrition experiments and experiences, (4) out-of-class experiences, and (5) academic controversies.[4] Competitive and individual learning are not as effective.

In cooperative learning, learners work together to achieve goals for learning that are mutually held. They collaborate, effectively share information and analyses, and teach and assist each other. By teaching others, a person enhances his own learning. A second strategy, inquiry learning, requires use of the problem-solving process, which consists of stating a problem, gathering data, analysing data, selecting possible solutions, testing solutions, and finally selecting the best solution to the problem. Clients can be guided through this process so that they learn to solve their own nutrition problems. Experiments using laboratory animals for nutrition research and hands-on activities, such as planning nutritious menus and preparing varieties of new foods for a diet, are a third approach. An example of using experiences outside of the classroom as a means of instruction is to require learners to shop for and evaluate certain foods. In using academic controversies, participants take opposing sides of an issue, explore their differences, and try to come to a consensus. These five types of experiences promote more elaborate cognitive processing, higher-level reasoning, problem solving, decision making, positive attitudes, and motivation. They can lead to group decisions in which members commit themselves publicly to better food habits.[4]

Modeling is another method of influencing behavior.[4,5] People learn by imitating others in unfamiliar or new situations. The instructor should behave as the learner is expected to behave, modeling the desirable attitude or behavior. People are more likely to accept new behaviors when they meet and have discussions with people who have successfully adopted them. This technique is appropriate for nutrition education.

Skills in the psychomotor domain are learned with direct experience and practice over time. The professional may begin with a demonstration, but then the learner needs to practice the skill under supervision. Coaching is a term that describes the assistance given to someone learning a new skill, and it can apply to an educational experience as well as a sport. It suggests a one-on-one, continuous, supportive relationship from which an individual learns over time. It is perhaps the best method of on-the-job training of employees. The trainer can give encouragement, confidence, and guidance as the trainee performs the task.[6] Coaching takes into consideration different learning abilities and needs, allows actual practice, and provides the person with immediate feedback regarding his performance.

TASK ANALYSIS

In instruction that requires the learner to develop a skill, a task analysis is helpful. An employee needs to learn the skills related to his job, and a client may need to develop skill in menu planning and food preparation using his new diet. Regardless of the kind of skill involved, the learner needs to be able to perform the skill initially, and then to improve the skill through continued practice. After mastering the basics of tennis, driving a car, or baking a cake, for example, the learner requires repeated experience to develop the skill.

Instruction involving the initial development of a skill requires an examination of what the job or task entails, the conditions under which it is performed, and the proper method of performance. The task should be broken down into its elements and key points and put into writing. If available, a job description may be used as a starting point in determining job content, but job descriptions do not give specific enough information for determining the content of training.[7] All of the tasks included in a job should be listed individually. If the job description is unavailable or incomplete, it may be necessary to interview the employee or observe his work to determine the job content. A waitress, for example, completes a number of tasks during the day, such as greeting customers, taking their orders, placing orders in the kitchen, serving the courses of the meal, busing dishes, setting tables, receiving payment for services, and maintaining good public relations. Each is a separate task contributing to the total job, and each task or set of actions can be defined.

The next step is to complete a written task analysis or series of task analyses for each different task of the job. A task analysis, sometimes referred to as a job breakdown, is a sequential list of the steps involved in performing any task from start to finish. Usually, the major steps are numbered, and each step describes what to do.[7] Many job-related tasks involve the psychomotor domain; thus, actions are listed in the analysis. It is often necessary, however, to have some background knowledge from the cognitive domain in performing the task. Balancing a checkbook, for example, is both a motor and intellectual skill, as is operating a cash register.

After the sequential steps are listed, each one should be examined to see whether there are explanations from the cognitive domain that need to be added. For example, if step one is to plug in the meat slicer, a key point is to have dry hands to avoid the danger of electrical shock. If a final step in the waitress's task analysis for busing dirty dishes includes washing hands, an explanation may be added regarding the transfer of microorganisms to clean food and utensils. In food service, sanitation and safety statements are frequently needed. Explanations of how or why a step is necessary or notes on materials or equipment may be considered. There are several different ways to complete a task analysis.[6–10]

Once written, the task analysis should be used by both the instructor and the learner. The instructor or trainer may examine the task analysis to construct learning objectives, which describe the behavior expected at the end of training. In assessing the learner's need for instruction, the instructor should consider the difference between the skill described in the task analysis and the learner's current skill to define the gap in knowledge or skill that must be addressed. The trainer should demonstrate to the individual what to do, and then allow him to perform the task. The learner may use the task analysis as a reference since it describes what to do in sequence. Using the task analysis in coaching or in supervised on-the-job training facilitates the learning of skills.

After mastering the basic skill and being able to recognize the correct sequence of procedures, the learner needs repeated practice to improve the skill. With time and practice, improvements in speed and quality of work should develop.

JOB INSTRUCTION TRAINING

A great deal of employee training takes place not in the classroom but on the job. New employees require orientation and training with either an experienced worker or a supervisor. Current employees may need retraining periodically, may be assigned new tasks, or may receive promotions, which require the development of new skills and abilities. During World War II when men left for the military services, there was a great need to train job replacements. A four-step process entitled Job Instruction Training (JIT) was delineated for rapid training of new employees. It was succesfully then, and with refinements, continues to be one means of training. It may be used to teach skills and is based on performance rather than subject matter. The four steps are preparation, presentation, learner performance, and follow-up. Prior to instruction, a task analysis should be completed, and the work area arranged with the necessary supplies and materials that the employee is expected to maintain.[8] JIT is outlined in the following:[8]

How to Instruct

Part I: Prepare the learner.

   Put him at ease.
   State the job.
   Find out what he knows about the job.
   Get him interested.
   Correct his position.

Part II: Present the operation.

   Tell, show, and illustrate.
   Explain one important step at a time.
   Stress key points.
   Instruct clearly, completely, and patiently, but no more than
      the learner can master.
   Summarize the operation in a second run-through.

Part III: Try out performance.

   Have learner do the job.
   Have learner explain key points as he does the job again.
   Make sure that he understands.
   Continue until you know that he knows the job.

Part IV: Follow up.

   Put learner on his own.
   Designate where to obtain help.
   Encourage questions.
   Taper off.
   Continue with normal supervision.

Part I of JIT prepares the employee psychologically and intellec-tually for learning. Since a superior may be the trainer, any tension, nervousness, or apprehension in the subordinate employee must be overcome, since it may interfere with learning. A friendly, smiling trainer puts the person at ease by creating an informal atmosphere for learning, where mistakes are expected and tolerated. He states the job to be learned and asks specific questions to determine what the learner already knows about it. If the employee becomes interested in the job, his motivation for learning increases. Finally, the trainer should be sure that the employee can physically see what is being demonstrated.

In Part II, the trainer presents and explains the operation as the employee will be expected to perform it. He tells, shows, and illustrates the operation one step at a time using a prepared task analysis. Key points should be stressed. The instruction should be carried out clearly, completely, and patiently, with the trainer remembering the employee's abilities and attitudes. Since the ability to absorb new information is limited, the trainer needs to determine how much the learner can master at one time. It may be 5 to 10 steps with key points, or it may be more. It may be 15 minutes or one hour of instruction. Overloading the learner with information is ineffectual since the information will be forgotten. After this initial instruction, the operation or task should be summarized and performed a second time.

Part III tests how much the learner has retained as he tries out the operation using the written task analysis as a reference. The learner does the job while the trainer or coach stands by to assist. Accuracy, not speed, is stressed initially. As the employee completes the task a second time, the trainer should ask him to state the key points. To be sure that the employee understands, the trainer should ask such questions as "What would happen if ... ?" "What else do you do ... ?" and "What next ... ?" The employee repeats the operation five times, ten times, or however many times are needed until he knows what to do. The trainer continues coaching and giving positive feedback, encouragement, and reassurance until the employee learns the operation.

Follow-up occurs in Part IV as supervision tapers off. At first, the employee is put on his own to complete the task. He should always know, however, where to obtain assistance if it is needed. Any additional questions ought to be encouraged since minor points may still arise. Normal supervision continues to ensure that the task is done as instructed, since fellow workers may suggest short cuts that are undesirable.

Mager has pointed out that when the learner's experience is followed by positive consequences, the individual will be stimulated to approach the situation, but that when aversive consequences follow, the learner will avoid the situation.[5] A positive consequence may be a pleasant event, praise, a successful experience, an increase in self-esteem, improvement in self-image, or an increase in confi-

dence. Aversive conditions are events or emotions that cause physical or mental discomfort, or that lead to loss of self-respect. They
include fear, anxiety, frustration, humiliation, embarrassment, and
boredom. In influencing learners in the affective domain as well as
in the other domains, the instructor should positively reinforce
learner responses.

SEQUENCE OF INSTRUCTION

Sequence of instruction is characterized by the progressive development of knowledge, attitudes, and skills. Learning takes place
over time, and the process should be organized into smaller units.
Since the ultimate outcome is able performance, it is important to
consider how meaningful the sequence is to the learner, not the
teacher, and whether or not it promotes learning. Mager provides
several recommendations for sequencing. Instruction may be arranged from the general to the specific, from the specific to the
general, from the simple to the complex, or according to interest,
logic, or frequency of use of the knowledge or skill.[9]

In moving from the general to the specific, an overview or large
picture should be presented first, and then the details and specifics
are presented. For example, an overview of the reasons for the
diabetic diet and the general principles of the diet should be presented prior to the details. With a new employee, a general explanation of the job should precede the specifics. Once the learner has
digested some information, it is possible to consider a specific to
general sequence.

Material may be organized from the simple (terms, facts, procedures) to the complex (concepts, processes, theories, analyses, applications) so that the learner handles increasingly difficult material.
If the taxonomies have been used in writing objectives for learning,
the hierarchy of the taxonomies provides a simple to complex sequence.

Another possibility is sequencing according to interest, or from
the familiar to the unfamiliar. One may begin instruction with whatever is of most interest or concern to the learner. An initial question
from the learner suggests such interest and should be dealt with
immediately so that he is free to concentrate on later information.
"How long will I have to stay on this diet?" "Can I eat my favorite
foods?" Information desired by the learner is a good starting point
for discussion. Similarly, if the learner perceives a problem, the
dietitian can start with his problem rather than with a preset agenda.
As learning proceeds, the individual may develop additional needs
for information or goals for learning, which they may then address.
Individuals who have assisted in directing their own learning tend
to feel more committed to it.

Logic may suggest the sequence. Certain things may need to be said before others. Safety precautions may need to be introduced early, for example, when discussing equipment. Sanitary handling of utensils may be important to discuss with a waitress prior to discussing how to set a table.

Frequency of use of the knowledge or skill may dictate sequence. The skill used more frequently should be taught first, followed by the next most frequently used skill. If training time runs out, at least the learner has learned all except the least frequently used skills.

Finally, the instructor should provide the learner with total job practice. While the learner may have been practicing individual elements of the job, he also needs to practice the total job. This practice may be provided in the actual job situation or through simulation.

EVALUATION OF RESULTS

The step most often overlooked in education is probably that of evaluation. The literature indicates that evaluation of nutrition programs is frequently omitted.[11] Evaluation connotes the determination of the value or worth of something. Everyone uses this process daily, both consciously and unconsciously. "Does the food taste good?" "Is he dressed well?" "Was the television show worth watching?" "Did I learn anything?" One's thoughts turn to evaluation automatically. According to Popham, systematic educational evaluation "consists of a formal assessment of the worth of educational phenomena."[12] That it is systematic suggests that advance planning has taken place and that the process will provide data on the merit of the educational endeavor.

Although the terms "measurement" and "evaluation" are frequently interchanged, their meanings should not be confused. Measured is the process of collecting and quantifying data on the extent, degree, or capacity of achievement. It is the act of determining the degree to which an individual possesses a certain attribute, as when he receives a score of 85 on a test, but it does not determine worth. Measurement systems require experimental designs, data collection, and statistical analysis of the data.[12] Evaluation goes beyond measurement to the formation of value judgments about the data. It may involve the use of criteria.

Purpose of Evaluation

There are several purposes of evaluation. Evaluation is a system of quality control to determine whether the process of education is effective, to identify its strengths and weaknesses, and to determine what changes should be made. It is important to determine whether the objectives were accomplished, and whether the individual learned what was intended or developed in desired ways.[13] Evaluation is helpful in making decisions concerning teaching, learning, program effectiveness, and the necessity of making modifications in current efforts or even of terminating them. In times of limited financial resources, accountability requires an examination of cost/benefit ratios. Is the program so useful and valuable that costs are justified? Evaluation provides evidence that what one is doing is worthwhile. Plans for evaluation should be made early when one is in the planning stages of an educational endeavor, and not after the endeavor has begun or is completed.

As with other parts of his adult education model, Knowles has suggested that evaluation should be a mutual undertaking between the educator and the learner.[14] He recommends less emphasis on the evaluation of learning, and more on the rediagnosis of learning needs, which will suggest immediate or future steps to be taken jointly by the professional and the learner. This type of feedback from evaluation is more constructive and more acceptable to adults. Thus, evaluation may be considered something one should do with people, not to people. If problems are apparent, then solutions may be found jointly by the educator and learner.

Formative and Summative Evaluation

Formative and summative evaluation are two types of evaluation used to improve any of three processes—curriculum construction, teaching, or learning. Formative evaluation refers to that made during the course of education, with the feedback of results guiding the rest of the educational endeavor. Summative evaluation refers to a summary assessment of results at the conclusion of learning.[15]

Formative evaluation is a systematic appraisal that occurs during a course of instruction or learning activity for the purpose of improving teaching or learning. It can help to diagnose problems in student learning and in teaching effectiveness. It pinpoints parts mastered and parts not mastered and allows for revision of plans, methods, techniques, or materials. Formative evaluation may be performed at frequent intervals. If the learner appears bored, unsure, anxious, quizzical, or lost, or if one is unsure of the person's abilities, stop teaching and start the evaluation process. Ask him to repeat what he has learned. In diabetic education, for example, if formative evaluation shows that the individual does not understand the concept of food exchange lists, he will not be able to master more complex behaviors, such as menu planning. Having located the problem that the exchange lists are not comprehended, the dietitian can change approaches to try to overcome the problem. Perhaps the use of an alternative explanation that is clearer or simpler, or the use of concrete illustrations, is indicated. Ideas and concepts may need to be reviewed. Sometimes, in group education, a group member is able to provide an explanation that the person understands better than the professional's explanation.

Failure to learn may not always be related to instructional methods or materials per se, but may derive from problems that are physical, emotional, cultural, or environmental in nature. By performing evaluations after smaller units of instruction, one can determine whether the pacing of instruction is appropriate for the patient or employee. Frequent feedback is necessary to facilitate learning. It is especially important when a great deal has to be learned. Mastery of smaller units can be a powerful positive reinforcement for the learner, and verbal reward may increase motivation to continue learning. When mistakes are made, they should be corrected quickly by giving the correct information. Avoid saying: "No, that's wrong." "Can't you ever get things right?" "Won't you ever learn?" Positive, not negative, feedback should be given. Approach the problem by saying, "Let me help you with that."

Summative evaluation has a different purpose and time frame than formative evaluation. Summative evaluation is considered final, and it is used at the end of a term, course, or learning activity. The purpose of summative evaluation may be grading, certification, or evaluation of progress, and the evaluation distinguishes those who excel from those who do not. Judgment is made about the learner, teacher, or curriculum with regard to the effectiveness of learning or instruction. This judgmental aspect creates the anxiety and defensiveness often associated with evaluation.

Evaluation should be a continuous process that is preplanned along with educational sessions. Evaluation preassessment determines the individual's abilities before the educational program, and progress should be evaluated continuously during as well as immediately following the educational program. Follow-up evaluation at three months or six months may measure the degree to which one has forgotten knowledge or has fallen back to previous behaviors.

Types of Evaluation

After considering the purpose and timing of evaluation, one should resolve the question of what to evaluate. Four types of evaluation have been suggested. These are (1) participant reactions to programs, (2) measures of organizational change, (3) measures of behavioral change, and (4) evaluation of learning.[13,16]

Participant Reaction. The first type of evaluation deals with participant reactions to educational programs. Did participants like the program, subject matter, content, materials, speakers, room arrangements, and learning activities? When a program, meeting, or class is evaluated, the purpose is to improve decisions concerning its various aspects, or to see how its parts fit the whole. These aspects may include structure, arrangements, administration, physical facilities, and personnel. The quality of such learning elements as objectives, techniques, materials, and learning outcomes may be included also. Hedonistic scales have been used to determine a happiness index, or the degree to which participants liked various aspects of the program. These judgments are subjective.

Organizational Change. Educators involved with employee training gather a second type of evaluative data to justify the time and expense to the organization. Management may want to know how training will benefit the organization. Results in terms of the following aspects may be attributed, at least in part, to training: employee turnover, frequency of accidents, absenteeism and attendance records, quality and quantity of product produced, dollar savings, number of employee errors, number of grievances, amount of overtime, employee productivity, and morale.

Behavioral Change. A third type of evaluation is the measurement of behavior. Did behavior or habits change based on the learning? In employee training, for example, one may assess changes in job behaviors to see whether transfer of training to the job has occurred. It is necessary to know what job performance was prior to training and to decide who will observe or assess changed performance—the supervisor, peers, or the individual. The ultimate aim of patient and client education is not merely the improvement in knowledge, but changes in dietary behaviors and practices. These changes are difficult to confirm and often depend on self-reports.

Learning. Whether learning has taken place is a separate question, even if the program rated highly on entertainment value. The learning of principles, facts, attitudes, values, and skills should be evaluated on an objective basis, and this task is more complex. If the learning objectives have been written in terms of measurable performance, they serve as the source of the evaluation. To what degree were the objectives achieved by the learner? Whether one has succeeded in learning can be determined by developing situations, or test items, based on the objectives of instruction. It is important for the test items to match the objectives in performance and conditions. If they do not match the objectives, it is not possible to assess whether instruction was successful, i.e., whether the learner learned what was intended.

Mager pointed out that there are a number of obstacles to overcome to assess the results of instruction successfully. Some obstacles are caused by the objectives, while others result from attitudes and beliefs on the part of instructor.[17]

One of the problems in evaluation results from inadequately written objectives. If the performance is not stated, if conditions are omitted, and if the criterion is missing, it will be difficult to create a test situation. If these deficiencies are discovered, the first step is to rewrite the objective.

Norm- and Criterion-Referenced Methods. The attitudes and beliefs of the instructor also influence the evaluation of learning. Some
attitudes may result from one's own experiences in school. One may
believe that the test should not be too easy, but the degree of
difficulty of a test is not important. The question is whether the
learner can perform what is stated in the objectives. Perhaps the
instructor believes that some of the questions have to be difficult
so that a spread in scores is produced, to separate the brightest
from the rest, the "A's" from the "B's" and "C's." Tests are purposely
developed so that not everyone will be successful. Students are
graded in a norm-referenced manner by comparison with others or
with the norm of the group. A norm-referenced instrument indicates
whether the individual's performance falls in the 50th percentile or
the 90th percentile in relation to the group norm.[12,17]

Another approach to evaluation is the criterion-referenced
method. Instead of comparing learners with each other, the instructor compares them with an objective standard of what the learner
is expected to know or to be able to perform. A criterion- referenced
measurement ascertains the person's status in respect to a defined
objective or standard, and test items correspond to the objectives.
If the learner can perform what is called for in the objective, the
learner has been successful. If not, criterion-referenced testing,
which tends to be more diagnostic, will indicate what is lacking,
and more learning can be planned.[12] No doubt everyone has had
the experience of being told to learn one thing and then being tested
on another. Instruction should benefit the learner, not the teacher.
What is important should be made known to the learner so that his
time and effort are not wasted. Well-written performance objectives
accomplish this. They should be used as the basis for assessing the
results of instruction. If everyone does well on the evaluation, the
instruction has been successful.[17]

Mager suggested a series of steps to select appropriate test
items:[17]

1. Match the performance and conditions of the test item to
   those of the objective.
2. Check whether the performance is a main intent or an
   indicator.
3. If the performance is an indicator, note the main intent.
   Note whether the performance is covert or overt.
4. Test for the indicator in objectives containing one.

The first step is to see whether the performance specified in the
test item is the same as that specified in the objective. If they do
not match, the test item must be revised, since it will not indicate
whether the objective has been accomplished. If the objective states

that the performance is "to plan menus," or "to operate the dish-washing machine," the test should involve planning menus or operating the dishwashing machine. It would be inappropriate to ask the learner to discuss the principles of writing menus or to label the parts of the dishwashing machine on a diagram.

In addition to matching performance, the test should use the same specific circumstances or conditions that are specified in the objective.

Example: (Given the disassembled parts of the meat slicer) is able to reassemble the parts in correct sequence.

The condition is "given the disassembled parts of the meat slicer." The instructor should provide a disassembled machine and ask the learner to reassemble it. An inappropriate test would be to ask the learner to list the steps in reassembling the meat slicer, or to discuss the safety precautions to be taken.

If the learner must perform under a range of conditions, it may be necessary to test performance using the entire range. If a client eats at home and in restaurants, the dietitian must determine whether he is capable of the particular dietary practice in both environments. If a student is learning to take a diet history, he should be taught to handle the range of conditions, including people of different age, socioeconomic, and ethnic groups. Not every condition can be taught and tested, but the common conditions that the learner will encounter should be included in the objectives and in testing.

The main intent of an objective may be stated clearly or it may be implied. The main intent is the performance, while an indicator is an activity through which the main intent is inferred.

Example: (Given in a copy of a sodium-restricted diet) is able to plan a menu for a complete day.

The main intent is to discriminate between foods permitted and omitted on the diet, and the indicator is the ability to plan menus. One infers that if accurate sodium-restricted menus are planned, the learner knows what is permitted and what is not. One should test for the indicator in objectives that contain one.

Some performances are overt, and others are covert. Overt actions are visible or audible, such as writing, verbally describing, and assembling. If the performance is overt, determine whether the test item matches the objective.

Example: Is able to reassemble the parts of the meat slicer.

The employee should be provided with the parts of the meat slicer and asked to reassemble them. Performance tests are appropriate when skills are taught. If the employee is being taught to use equipment, the evaluation should be to have him demonstrate its operation. If a student is learning interviewing skills, an interview session is indicated as the evaluation. Covert actions are not visible, but are internal or mental activities, such as solving problems or identifying. If the performance is covert, an indicator should have been added to the objective as explained in Chapter 7, and the indicator should be tested.

Example: Is able to identify the parts of the meat slicer (on a diagram or verbally).

For this example, the learner should be provided with the indicator, a diagram of a meat slicer, and asked to identify the parts.

The discussion to this point has used examples of objectives in the cognitive and psychomotor domains. Affective objectives describe values, interests, and attitudes. While the cognitive and psychomotor domains are concerned with what an individual can do, the affective domain is concerned with what he is willing to do. These changes are covert or internal, may develop more slowly over a period of time. Evaluation of their achievement is more difficult and may need to take different forms. To assess whether the learner has been influenced by education, the professional may conduct discussion and listen to what the learner says or observe what he does, since both saying and doing are overt behaviors. To evaluate change in the learner's behavior, the evaluator attempts to secure data that permit an inference to be made regarding the learner's future disposition in similar situations. In the affective domain, this task is more difficult.

It is conceivable that the learner may display a desirable overt behavior only in the presence of the instructor. The attitude toward following a diabetic diet or an employee work procedure may differ, depending on the dietitian's presence or absence. Since time is required for change in the affective domain, evaluation may have to be repeated at designated intervals. To determine realistically how the person is disposed to act, the measurement approach needs to evoke volitional rather than coerced responses.

Other outcomes of nutrition education may be measures of nutritional status, such as weight loss; change in clinical or biochemical indices, such as serum cholesterol level in cardiovascular disease, hemoglobin level in pregnancy, and glycosylated hemoglobin level in diabetes; or reduction in risk factors for disease and improved health, both of which are long-term goals. Care must be taken in interpreting some of these results since they may reflect other variables besides education. For example, stress can affect one's blood sugar even when the diabetic diet is followed.[18]

Data Collection Techniques

There are a number of techniques for collecting evaluation data. They include paper-and-pencil tests, questionnaires, interviews, visual observation, job sample or performance tests, simulation, rating forms or checklists, individual and group performance measures, individual and group behavior measures, and self-reports.[13,19] As measurement devices that will be analyzed statistically, they require the use of specific experimental designs. Regardless of the particular technique used, it should be pretested with a smaller group prior to actual use. Since comparisons are desired, it is usually necessary to collect preliminary data on current performance or behaviors.

Tests, especially written tests, are probably the most common devices for measuring learning. Schools depend heavily on them, and as a result, they are familiar to everyone. Multiple-choice, true-false, short-answer, completion, matching, and essay questions are used to measure learning in the cognitive domain.[15] These tests are often used when several people are expected to learn the same content or material. Sometimes, both a pretest and a posttest are used to measure learning. This method assists in controlling variables, but one should be careful not to attribute all of the change noted on the posttest to the learning experiences, since other factors may have been involved.[12] In a child's school experiences, the teacher assigns grades based on test scores. With adults, the educator should avoid evoking childhood memories associated with the authoritarian teacher, the dependent child, or the assigned degrees of success or failure. In one-on-one situations, the educator may ask the learner to state verbally what he has learned as though he were telling it to a spouse or friend.

Questionnaires may be preplanned and are often used to assess attitudes and values, which do not involve correct answers. Questions may be open-ended, multiple-choice, ranking, checklist, or alternate-response, such as yes/no or agree/disagree.

Interviews conducted on a one-to-one basis are another form of evaluation. They are the oral equivalent to written questionnaires used to measure cognitive and affective objectives. Prior to the interview, the evaluator should draw up a list of questions that will indicate whether learning has taken place. After instruction, evaluation may consist of asking the client or employee to repeat important facts. An advantage of an interview is that the evaluator can put the person at ease and immediately correct any errors. Another advantage is that the interviewer can probe for additional information. Although this method is time-consuming, it is appropriate for the illiterate or less educated.

In many cases, visual observation is an appropriate method of evaluating learning. The behaviors to be observed should be defined, and an observation checklist may be helpful. When employees are under direct supervision, systematic ongoing observation over a period of time is a basis for evaluating learning. The professional can observe whether the employee is operating equipment correctly or following established procedures properly. If the employee has been taught sanitary procedures, for example, the professional can see whether or not they are incorporated into the employee's work. One should evaluate the performance, using what was taught as a standard. If discrepancies are found, further learning may be indicated.

Where direct observation is not possible or would be too time-consuming, a simulated situation or performance test can be observed. Performance tests are appropriate in the cognitive and psychomotor domains. One could ask a waitress to set a table, a cook to demonstrate the meat slicer, or a client to indicate what to select from a restaurant menu. The patient could be given a list of foods, some of which are permitted on the diet and some of which are not, and asked to differentiate them. Audiotape or videotape may be utilized to record the simulation, so that the instructor and learner may discuss the results together and plan further learning to correct any deficiencies. The learner should give permission in advance if taping is to be used. The observer needs to delineate which behaviors are being observed and what is to be considered acceptable behavior.

Rating scales or checklists have been used to evaluate learner performance and teacher effectiveness. Categories or attributes, such as knowledge level or dependability, are listed, and these should be defined in detail to avoid ambiguity. Emphasis should be placed on attributes that can be confirmed objectively rather than judged subjectively. A five- or seven-point scale is used, allowing a midpoint, and the range should be defined, e.g., from "excellent" to "poor" or from "extremely acceptable" to "very unacceptable." The list should include as a possible response, "No opportunity to observe."

Rating scales are subject to a number of errors. Two evaluators may judge the same individual differently. To avoid error, definition of the terms and training of evaluators are essential. The ratings may suffer from personal bias. In addition, some raters have the tendency to be too lenient. Error may also result if the rater is a perfectionist. Some evaluators tend to rate most people as average, believing that few people rank at the highest levels. Another possible error is the "halo effect," in which an evaluator is so positively or negatively impressed with one aspect of an individual that he judges all other qualities of the individual according to this one impressive aspect.

In employee training programs, individual and group performance measures, such as work quality, work quantity, and number of errors, may be assessed. Individual and group behavioral measures, such as amount of absenteeism, number of grievances, and other types of nonperformance problems that affect work performance, may be noted.

Self-reports are another approach to evaluation. In the affective domain, written questions or statements are presented, and the individual supplies responses. Responses may be distorted if the learner can ascertain the socially acceptable answer. Role-playing, simulation, and attitudinal scales have also been utilized. Self-reports such as a three-day food record have also been used to measure behavioral change, and in the Multiple Risk Factor Intervention Trial (MRFIT), a food score was developed, permitting participants to score their own food choice.[20]

All methods of evaluation have advantages and limitations, which need to be considered. In assessing adult learning, the evaluator should be careful to protect the individual's self-concept and to treat errors as indications for additional instruction.

Reliability/Validity

The concepts of reliability and validity are important to the measurement of learning. Validity indicates whether a test measures what it is designed to measure. There are different types of validity, such as content, construct, concurrent, and predictive validity, which help to "defend" the validity of the instrument. Content validity, which is probably the most important for criterion-referenced testing, refers to whether the test items correspond to the content of instruction. Reliability refers to the consistency with which a test or device measures something over time. For example, if a test is given twice to the same students to sample the same abilities, the students should place in the same relative position to others each time if the test is reliable. Methods for determining the reliability and validity of tests may be found in the educational literature.[12] In all cases, one must keep in mind that the test or measuring device should assess whether the learner has attained the requisite knowledge, skill, or competence needed. If the learner has not attained the intended knowledge or skill, additional learning may be indicated.

Once the data from evaluation have been collected, they should be compiled and analyzed. The statistical analysis of data that is required is a lengthy subject of its own and is beyond the scope of this book. Future plans or programs may be modified based on the results of the evaluation. Results should be communicated to such others as participants, top management staff, decision makers, and future learners.

LESSON PLANS

A lesson plan is a written summary of information about a unit of instruction. It is prepared and used by the instructor and may be submitted to an administrator. Various formats for lesson plans are available, but the content for each is essentially the same.

A lesson plan describes all aspects of instruction. It includes the plans for preassessment; the objectives; the content and how it will be sequenced; a description of the activities that learners will engage in to reach the objectives; instructional procedures, materials, teaching aids, media, and equipment to be used; the amount of time alloted; facilities to be used; and a method of evaluating whether the learner has reached the objectives.[9] Once written, a lesson plan is a flexible guide to instruction that can be used with many different individuals or groups. A series of lesson plans may be grouped into a larger unit of instruction.

DOCUMENTATION

Dietitians are accountable for the nutritional care they provide. Accepted standards of practice and accreditation agencies mandate that dietetic services be documented for review. Documentation has been described as "the method by which others are made aware of specific approaches to client problems and outcomes," and it provides a "developmental history" of nutritional services to clients.[11] What takes place between the dietitian and the client should be recorded, including nutritional assessment, nutrition care plans, goals, means of achieving goals and their outcomes, nutritional counseling and education, as well as where efforts ought to be directed in the future. The information communicated demonstrates what the nutrition professional contributes to health care delivery.

The usual place for documentation is the client's record. Frequently, the dietitian makes notes on the patient's medical record using the SOAP procedure. The acronym SOAP stands for Subjective data, Objective data, Assessment, and Plan. Subjective data include the client's perception and thoughts about the nutrition problem and his food intake. Objective data are the results of laboratory tests, such as serum albumin, or physical findings, such as weight or height. Assessment is the dietitian's analysis of the person's problem based on the subjective and objective data. The Plan tells what the dietitian recommends or intends to do to solve a particular problem, such as plans for patient counseling, education, or other follow-up practices.[21]

Documentation of employee education and training programs is also essential. Records should be kept of all material included in employee orientation. The use of an orientation checklist is helpful in ensuring that everything the employee needs to know has been communicated to him. Records should be kept on file showing the date and content of ongoing training sessions such as inservice programs, and of off-the-job experiences such as continuing education.

This chapter has examined the selection and implementation of learning activities in the cognitive, affective, and psychomotor domains. The use of a task analysis and job instruction training for learning the psychomotor domain have been explained. The final step in planning learning is evaluation, in which data are collected and analyzed to determine the success of educational endeavors.

The educator seeks to influence behavior by imparting information to learners. The nutrition educator seeks to change people's eating practices, and the employee trainer seeks to change the employee's job performance. Techniques and strategies that influence the acquisition of knowledge, the development of appropriate attitudes, and behavioral change have been discussed. The relationship of knowledge and attitudes to behavior is complex, however, since behavior is subject to many motivations, all operating at the same time. The fact that clients or employees are informed does not mean that they will always act intelligently. Motives may be conflicting, and information may be disregarded or altered to serve one's own purposes.[4] If time is limited, for example, little thought may be given to food choices. Instructional techniques that promote interpersonal interaction and reflect the social context are important influences in nutrition education.

SUGGESTED ACTIVITIES

1. Complete a task analysis for using a procedure or a piece of equipment, listing the sequential steps and key points.

2. Using the Job Instruction Training sequence and a task analysis, teach someone to use a piece of equipment that is not familiar to them.

3. Plan learning using one of the techniques described in the chapter (other than lecture), such as discussion, simulation, or demonstration. Carry out the plan.

4. Develop one or two performance objectives on a topic of interest, and plan the content, techniques for presentation, teaching aids, and evaluation methods. Carry out the educational plan.

5. Give a pretest of knowledge on a subject. Instruct the learner on the subject. Follow up with a posttest.

6. List three ways in which one might evaluate whether an employee learned from a training program. List three ways in which one might

evaluate whether a patient comprehended instruction regarding a diabetic diet.

7. Identify which of the following is a norm-referenced test and which is a criterion-referenced test.

A. Learners are given a nationally administered test of knowledge, and individual scores are reported and compared.

B. Learners are given a test prepared by the teacher based on learning objectives.

Answers:

7A. Norm-referenced.

7B. Criterion-referenced.

REFERENCES

1. Hutchinson, D.: The process of planning programs of continuing education for health manpower. *In* Fostering the Growing Need to Learn. Rockville, MD, Division of Regional Medical Programs, 1973.
2. Spitz, H.: Choosing Techniques for Teaching and Learning. Washington, DC, National Education Assoc., 1970.
3. Craig, R. (ed.): Training and Development Handbook. 2nd ed. New York, McGraw-Hill, 1976.
4. Johnson, D.W., and Johnson, R.T.: Nutrition education: A model for effectiveness, a synthesis of research. J. Nutr. Ed., *17*:S1, 1985.
5. Mager, R.F.: Developing Attitudes Toward Learning. Palo Alto, CA, Fearon Publishers, 1968.
6. Rose, J.C.: Handbook for Health Care Food Service Management. Rockville, MD, Aspen Publications, 1984.
7. Wexley, K., and Latham, G.: Identifying training needs. *In* The Training and Development Sourcebook. Edited by L. Baird et al. Amherst, MA, Human Resource Development Press, 1983.
8. McCord, B.: Job instruction. *In* Training and Development Handbook. 2nd ed. Edited by R. Craig. New York, McGraw-Hill, 1976.
9. Mager, R.F., and Beach, K.M.: Developing Vocational Instruction. Belmont, CA, Fearon Publishers, 1967.
10. Laird, D., and House, R.: Training Today's Employees. Boston, CBI Publishing Co., 1983.
11. Wills, B.B.: Documentation: The missing link in evaluation. J. Am. Diet. Assoc., *85*:225, 1985.
12. Popham, W.J.: Educational Evaluaton. Englewood Cliffs, NJ, Prentice-Hall, 1975.
13. Phillips, J.J.: Handbook of Training Evaluation and Measurement Methods. Houston, Gulf Publishing Co., 1983.
14. Knowles, M.S.: The Adult Learner: A Neglected Species. 2nd ed. Houston, Gulf Publishing Co., 1978.
15. Bloom, B.S., Hastings, J.T., and Madaus, G.F.: Handbook on Formative and Summative Evaluation of Student Learning. New York, McGraw-Hill, 1971.
16. Kirkpatrick, D.: Evaluation of training. *In* Training and Development Handbook. 2nd ed. Edited by R. Craig. New York, McGraw-Hill, 1976.
17. Mager, R.F.: Measuring Instructional Intent or Got a Match? Belmont, CA, Lear Siegler Inc., 1973.
18. Fruin, M.F., and Davison, M.L.: Some considerations in the measurement of change. J. Am. Diet. Assoc., *73*:15, 1978.

19. Parker, T.: Statistical methods for measuring training results. *In* Training and Development Handbook. 2nd ed. Edited by R. Craig. New York, McGraw-Hill, 1976.
20. Remmell, P.S., Gorder, D.D., Hall, Y., and Tillotson, J.L.: Assessing dietary adherence in the Multiple Risk Factor Intervention Trial (MRFIT). J. Am. Diet. Assoc., *76*:351, 1980.
21. Mason, M., Wenberg, B.G., and Welsch, P.K.: The Dynamics of Clinical Dietetics. 2nd ed. New York, John Wiley and Sons, 1982.

9

Motivation

A major theme of this book has been the need for dietitians to motivate clients and staff. Motivation is important in setting goals, planning behavioral modification strategies, designing and executing educational curriculum or training seminars, counseling others individually or in groups, and defusing hostility or working through conflict situations. The dietitian who understands motivational concepts and has the skills to adapt them to particular situations significantly increases his chances for being professionally successful.

Motivation can be defined as something that causes a person to act. It can also refer to the process of stimulating a person to action. It is concerned with the question of why human behavior occurs. The word itself is frequently used "to describe those processes that (1) arouse and instigate behavior; (2) give direction and purpose to behavior; (3) continue to allow behavior to persist; and (4) lead to choosing or preferring a particular behavior."[1] It is concerned not only with what a person *can* do, but also with what he *will* do.

Individuals can be motivated in many ways. Some can motivate themselves, while others must be goaded, threatened, or challenged to act. Those in the first category are referred to as "motivation seekers" and are motivated primarily by the nature of the task or job they perform. Most people, however, need to be stimulated to act, particularly when a change in lifestyle, diet, or health practices is necessary.[2]

Motivation is complex, and there are a number of factors or variables, both intrinsic and extrinsic, that influence the process at any one moment in time. Today's motivational influences may differ from tomorrow's, and short-term goals may take precedence over the long-term ones. Having knowledge of how one should work to get the most accomplished, of what one should eat to become or remain healthy, or of what one should do to cope with a current physiological condition such as diabetes may easily be overpowered by other motivational factors. The problem is that being motivated to work, to become or remain healthy, or to learn what one needs for appropriate cardiovascular or diabetes care involves long-term goals, and eating something such as chocolate cake, or coming in late for work "just this once," meets a short-term goal of pleasure. Some people may delay the long-term for the immediate pleasure. Although there is a great deal of knowledge concerning motivation that is helpful, there are no "miracle methods or universal answers to difficult motivational problems."[1]

Motivation can arise from factors that are either intrinsic or extrinsic, and these factors can affect the individual either positively or negatively. Intrinsic motivation arises from within an individual, owing to his needs, desires, drives, or goals. An individual who desires to be promoted, for example, has internal goals that motivate his performance. A man who has recently suffered a heart attack may be intrinsically motivated to change his dietary practices. External or extrinsic factors may supplement intrinsic motivation positively, or they may serve as barriers having a negative impact on motivation. Examples of positive external factors enhancing motivation include support from others, praise, or material rewards. An individual's motivation toward achieving dietary goals, however, may be hampered by social occasions or by family or friends who are not supportive and offer improper foods.

Dietitians are involved daily in motivating employees and clients, and they need to understand this complicated concept and its multiple processes. The administrative dietitian influences the motivation of employees, who must learn the procedures necessary to work effectively, do their jobs conscientiously without close supervision, and grow to improve in the work environment. The clinical dietitian must motivate not only staff, but also clients, who may need to learn about such things as the effects of diet on prenatal care, or the problems of sodium, cholesterol, or sugar in the diet. After they have been motivated to learn and to appreciate their problem or situation cognitively, motivation becomes a factor in obtaining their participation in dietary counseling and compliance with a dietary regimen.

This chapter discusses motivation in the three contexts previously mentioned: as an aid to client compliance, as an aid to teaching, and as an aid to managing staff. Although these three areas are treated separately in the chapter, the same motivational principles and theories apply to all of them.

MOTIVATION OF CLIENTS AND PATIENTS

The aim of nutritional counseling and education is to change food and eating behaviors so that the individual selects a healthier diet. Food selection is a part of a complex behavioral system, which is shaped by a vast array of variables. The food selection of a child is determined primarily by his parents and by the cultural and ethnic practices of his group. Early experiences and continuing interactions with food determine the food preferences, habits, and attitudes exhibited by adults. In addition to the profound role of family and culture in making dietary choices, influences include price of food, prestige value of food, religion, geography, peer and social influences, advertising, facilities, food preparation and storage, skills of the consumer in food preparation, time factors and convenience, and personal preferences and tolerances. All of these factors make food consumption a highly individual matter and resistant to change.[3]

In spite of problems associated with changing food behaviors, some people do change. People today are consuming less red meat and eggs than previously, for example. A summary of some of the motivational forces that influence the eating practices of clients is presented in Figure 9-1. Practitioners and other health educators should consider these factors with their clients and possibly add others, from their own experience. More detailed discussions of some of the variables are found in previous chapters.

Knowledge of which foods to consume is a first step in influencing healthful food behaviors, but it is probably overrated. When people do not follow their diets, some health educators tend to devote more and more time to teaching, redoubling their efforts and assuming that the problem is a deficit in knowledge, rather than exploring other motivational factors that may be more important. The relationship between what a person knows and what he does or how he behaves has been described as a "highly tenuous one," with only a weak relationship, if any, between nutritional knowledge and dietary practices.[4] Knowledge does not instigate change, but functions as an instrument if and when people want to make changes.[5] Better educated people may rely more on facts and knowledge as motivators for changing behavior than those who are less educated.[4]

Other motivational factors, both intrinsic and extrinsic, may encourage changes in food behaviors. People's interest in health, and their beliefs regarding nutrition as a factor in health promotion and disease prevention, may affect food choices. For example, a health belief that food was "good for them" correlated strongly with dietary practices among older women, but less so for those among younger women.[3] Postive cognitions such as "Nutrition is important" and "This dietary change is worth the effort" are helpful. Since food's flavor, convenience, and cost are prime motivators of food choices, Hochbaum has suggested that a nutritious diet should offer these advantages, and that these aspects should be stressed more than potential health benefits.[5] Dietitians therefore, need to overcome the public's perception that nutritious diets are costly, insipid, and inconvenient to purchase and prepare. They must promote the perception that dietary changes are pleasurable and possible. Previous chapters have emphasized the importance of having clients set one or two short-term goals for change and have suggested the use of self-monitoring of food intake and written contracts.

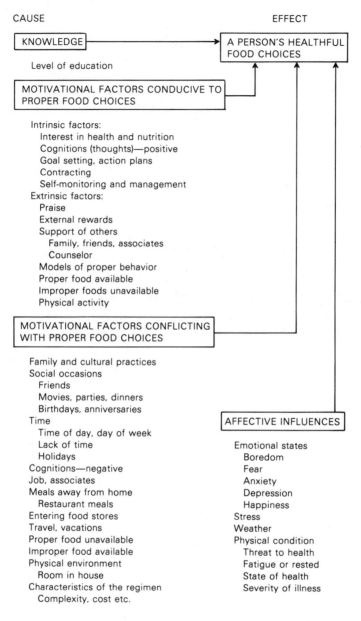

VARIABLES MOTIVATING CHANGE IN FOOD CHOICES AND HEALTH BEHAVIOR

CAUSE

EFFECT

KNOWLEDGE ──────────────▶ A PERSON'S HEALTHFUL FOOD CHOICES

Level of education

MOTIVATIONAL FACTORS CONDUCIVE TO PROPER FOOD CHOICES

Intrinsic factors:
    Interest in health and nutrition
    Cognitions (thoughts)—positive
    Goal setting, action plans
    Contracting
    Self-monitoring and management
Extrinsic factors:
    Praise
    External rewards
    Support of others
        Family, friends, associates
        Counselor
    Models of proper behavior
    Proper food available
    Improper foods unavailable
    Physical activity

MOTIVATIONAL FACTORS CONFLICTING WITH PROPER FOOD CHOICES

Family and cultural practices
Social occasions
    Friends
    Movies, parties, dinners
    Birthdays, anniversaries
Time   AFFECTIVE INFLUENCES
    Time of day, day of week
    Lack of time   Emotional states
    Holidays   Boredom
Cognitions—negative   Fear
Job, associates   Anxiety
Meals away from home   Depression
    Restaurant meals   Happiness
Entering food stores   Stress
Travel, vacations   Weather
Proper food unavailable   Physical condition
Improper food available   Threat to health
Physical environment   Fatigue or rested
    Room in house   State of health
Characteristics of the regimen   Severity of illness
    Complexity, cost etc.

Fig. 9-1. Variables motivating change in food choices and health behavior. A given behavior, such as choosing healthful foods, is affected by more factors than an individual's knowledge of what to do. Level of motivation is influenced by a number of interacting variables, which may differ on a daily basis.

Motivation provided by intrinsic factors may be supplemented by extrinsic factors. Praise and material rewards are positive consequences for proper food behaviors, and they may serve to enhance motivation. The support of significant others—family, friends, and the health counselor—is helpful. People who model proper skills can influence others to follow. Needless to say, healthful foods should be made readily available while improper foods should not. Alternative activities, such as physical activity, may also serve to promote change.

In spite of positive motivational and lifestyle factors, barriers to motivation may arise. Clients should be told to expect problems. The health educator should examine these problems with clients and attempt to reduce or eliminate them. Social occasions, holidays, eating in restuarants, weekend activities, food shopping, and travel require preplanning. A particular time of day, a particular day of the week, or just a lack of time may be barriers to healthful food choices. Problems may also arise from a person's workplace and job associates, and from not having the right foods available. Negative cognitions such as "It's not worth it" and "I'd rather die young and happy than follow this diet" interfere with motivation. Some people discover cues to improper eating in their physical environment, such as in certain rooms of the house. The characteristics of the regimen, such as complexity and cost, are other factors.

Food choices are also influenced by several affective factors involving attitudes, beliefs, and values. Attitudes are thought to be predispositions to action.[6] Such emotional states as boredom, anxiety, and depression may lead to eating the wrong food, but so may happiness and elation. Fear of illness or death can be a motivating factor, as can stress and the individual's physical condition. Whether the person is tired or rested, whether his medical problem is new or not, the severity of his illness, and its perceived threat to health may each influence motivation.

Motivation to make and maintain dietary changes is complex, for behavior is influenced by many motivational factors operating simultaneously. The interrelationships among knowledge, attitudes, and behavior are described as "more intricate than many of the studies of nutrition education acknowledge."[6] While knowledge of proper food choices is an essential first step in changing food behaviors, knowledge may be easily overpowered by something that seems more important at the moment. Following a proper diet to promote health and prevent disease is a long-term goal with rewards situated in the future, which may do little to enhance motivation. More immediate rewards may take precedence, such as eating a luscious piece of chocolate cake right now for the pleasure of it.

Nothing is known about the relative importance of each of the variables involved in motivation, the possible interaction of the factors, or the strength of their effect on food selection. Motivational variables directing today's food choices probably differ from tomorrow's and next week's choices, owing to changes in environmental dynamics. Behavioral change requires a major personal commitment, the setting of goals for change, support from others in one's efforts to modify long-standing practices, and reduction or elimination of barriers in the social, cultural, physical, and psychological environments of the individual. Although studies have focused on knowledge and attitude changes affecting eating practices, few studies have dealt with the complexity of all of the behaviors involved in food selection.[5]

MOTIVATION IN TEACHING

Teaching is a job responsibility of most dietitians, and nutrition education of the public is viewed as an obligation of all practitioners. The clinical dietitian may teach an individual or a group such subjects as proper nutrition practices for senior citizens, recommended prenatal nutrition, preparing nutritious meals on a limited budget, losing weight, and so forth. The administrative dietitian's teaching responsibilities include providing orientation for new employees, training staff in new practices and procedures, and coaching subordinates on a one-on-one basis. One of the keys to successful teaching is learner motivation.

Motivation is complicated and multifaceted. There is no single element that controls success. The best lesson plans, optimal materials, a well-informed and highly motivated dietitian-teacher, and an interesting and current curriculum cannot continuously guarantee that individuals will want to learn.[1]

Teachers do not motivate learners directly. They can make learning attractive and stimulating, however, provide opportunities and incentives, encourage the development of competence, and match the learner's interest with learning activities. Because there is no direct line of control between teacher behavior and individual motivation, the intervening variables of the learner's perceptions, values, personality, and judgments ultimately account for his degree of motivation.

This section is intended to enhance the dietitian's teaching and to facilitate learning by focusing on the practical use of knowledge about motivation. Though it is incomplete, the extant knowledge on motivation is considerable and can be applied logically and effectively through careful planning.

Time-Continuum Model of Motivation. Learning situations can be divided according to a three-period time continuum, consisting of a beginning, middle, and end, with motivation being facilitated during each of the stages through a motivational method.[1] Wlodkowski discusses the critical periods and the factors that can be applied to motivational strategies within each period (Fig. 9-2).[1]

The first critical period ("beginning") occurs when the learner enters the learning process. Two general motivational factors during this stage are (1) the learner's attitude toward the learning environment, teacher, subject matter, and self, and (2) his needs at the time of learning. Needs are experienced by the individual as forces moving him in the direction of a goal. The second period ("during") occurs when the person is involved in the body or main content of the learning process. The general motivational factors during this stage are (1) the stimulation process, which affects the individual as he becomes involved in the learning experience, and (2) the simultaneous affective or emotional experience of the learner. The third period ("ending") occurs when the person finishes or completes the learning process. The motivational factors during this stage are (1) the sense of competence developed from the person's learning experience and (2) the quality of the reinforcement that results from the learning experience.

To facilitate motivation, to prevent problems with motivation, and to diagnose potential for motivation in learning situations, the die-

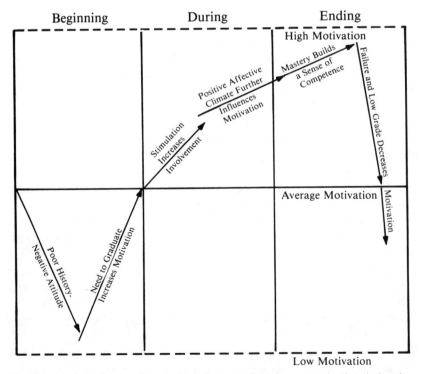

Fig. 9-2. Model indicating the relationships and influences on motivation during three time periods. (From Wlodkowski, R.J.: Motivation and Teaching. Washington, DC, National Education Assoc., 1984.)

titian needs to understand and evaluate the six factors described in the preceding paragraph as they occur during the critical time periods of a learning event. The following example is intended to illustrate how the multiple motivational factors interact on a dynamic basis to help or hinder motivation along a time continuum (see Fig. 9-2).

An indigent client may have had little success is working with health professionals and as a result may feel defensive and have a poor "attitude" toward the subject matter. This same individual, however, may "need" the information the dietitian has to share to feed his family well on a limited budget; thus, he may feel some sense of determination to complete the program. At this beginning stage, the dietitian has a client who is not enthusiastic but is willing to "give it a try." If the professional provides material and experiences that are interesting and appropriate, the client may find the class "stimulating" and sincerely try to do well. If he enjoys the other participants in the program, and if they work well together in solving mutual problems, he may become even more motivated by the "affective" climate. At the end of the program, if the client feels that he has mastered the content and has a sense of confidence and "competence," he will feel encouraged or "reinforced," and will probably continue with this new interest in the future.

One might infer from Figure 9-2 that the three phases of motivational impact are independent of one another. Wlodkowski points out, however, that the motivational influence constantly interacts with the learner. At the end stage, for example, the competence and reinforcement value interact with the previous factors to affect the learner's motivation at the moment. This interaction results in new attitudes and needs.

Any single motivational factor can have an overwhelming influence on a particular learning situation. The negative influence of one factor may be so powerful that it prevents involvement in learning. Alternatively, the positive influence of a factor may be so strong that it produces a desire to learn that supersedes the possible negative influence of the other factors. For example, an employee with a negative attitude may refuse to try to learn even though he needs the skills presented in the training for future advancement. The negative attitude may prevail even though he has peers in the course whom he enjoys, has the ability to master the material that is presented in a stimulating way, and knows that he will receive a wage increase upon successful completion. Another employee, whose desire for future advancement is strong, may learn in spite of course material that he believes is useless, instructors whom he experiences as boring, and a sense of isolation between himself and his peers. In most instances, however, influence of the motivational factors is more equally distributed.

Because the dietitian generally does not know which of the six factors is going to be the most critical for individuals, he should plan strategies for each factor, providing continuous and interactive motivational dynamics (Fig. 9-3). Six basic questions useful in planning a learning experience are:

1. What can the instructor do to encourage a positive attitude toward the learning situation?
2. What can be done to satisfy an individual's needs through the learning activities?
3. Are there ways to stimulate the individuals continuously while they are learning?
4. What might increase the positive affective or emotional climate for this particular learning activity?

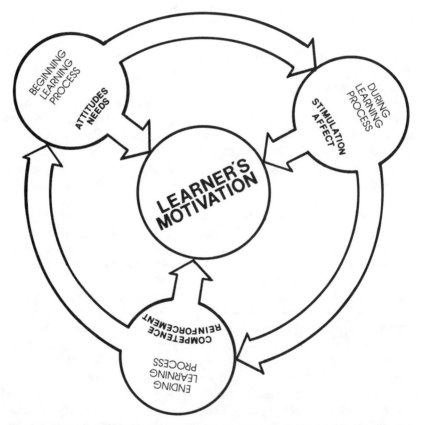

Fig. 9-3. Organizational aid to be applied to groups of individuals. When the dietitian attends to the six factors, he can, in any learning situation, design motivation strategies for his clients and staff throughout the learning process. (From Wlodkowski, R.J.: Motivation and Teaching. Washington, DC, National Education Association, 1984.)

5. How can this learning activity be structured to increase the person's feelings of competence?
6. What reinforcement will this activity provide?

MOTIVATION OF EMPLOYEES

This section explores the concept of motivation as it relates to employees and examines theories of motivation and their behavioral implications for dietitians. Although the concept of motivation was defined earlier in this chapter, the reader should keep in mind that motivational forces are usually multiple rather than singular, that they differ in strength, and that more than one may be present at a given time.

Maslow and Herzberg. Two theorists who have made major contributions to the study of motivation are Abraham Maslow and Frederick Herzberg. Maslow correlated human motivation with individual desires. In his "hierarchy of needs" theory and "need-priority" model, he lists five universal needs to explain human motivation: physiological needs; the need for safety and security; social needs; the need for esteem; and the need for self-realization (Fig. 9-4). For each need to become active as a motivating factor, the desire im-

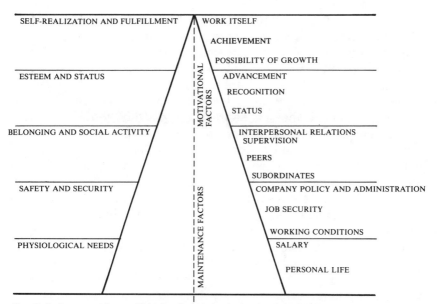

Maslow's Need—Priority Model   **Herzberg's Motivation—Maintenance Model**

Fig. 9-4. A comparison of Maslow's need-priority model with Herzberg's motivation-maintenance model. (Adapted from Herzberg, F.: Work and the Nature of Man. Cleveland, OH, World Publishing Co., 1966, and from Maslow, A.H.: Motivation and Personality. New York, Harper and Bros., 1954.)

mediately preceding the need must be fulfilled. In simplified terms, Maslow would say that the way to stimulate motivation in an individual is to determine which of his wants is most unsatisfied and then to structure his work so that in the accomplishment of the work goal, he satisfies his personal goals as well.[7] Wlodkowski has described Maslow's theory as being the most holistic and dynamic approach offering an interrelated set of guidelines to enhance learner motivation.[1]

The most basic human requirements are physiological. Sickness and hunger tend to take precedence over all other human needs. Only after they are satisfied does one experience the desire to satisfy the other needs. An indigent person who is able to take care of only his physiological necessities may work regardless of the working conditions for his own and his family's sustenance and shelter. Once he has enough money to satisfy these basic essentials, however, working merely for nourishment and shelter is no longer adequate. At that point, the individual's motivation to work arises from a drive to maintain safety and security. In most organizations today, these needs are satisfied through work contracts, unions, governmental regulations, and various insurance plans. With the fulfillment of biological and security needs, the individual's urge for social affiliation and activity becomes the dominant unsatisfied need, and it should therefore be considered in designing work goals to motivate the employee. Social needs can be experienced as a desire to become a member of, and participate in, a recognized group: family, church, community, work, neighborhood business, union, and so forth. Should this need become satiated, the employee's motivation is stimulated by his desire for esteem and status, which is commonly experienced as the need to attain recognition for accomplishments.

Although each of the five areas of needs becomes dominant at some time, the strongest motivator at a given moment is the one immediately above the last need satisified. Once the requirement for esteem is no longer lacking, for example, the desire for self-realization will become dominant. Self-realization is the highest human urge and the most self-centered. This drive for self-realization and the opportunity to grow as a person can be fulfilled only when most other needs are met. This need is commonly experienced as an urge for personal and professional growth through the work experience.

It is difficult for dietitians to apply Maslow's theory with any degree of certainty. Unless one has very few others reporting to him, the task of getting to know subordinates well enough to infer their current need level accurately is not likely to be accomplished; furthermore, need intensity at each level can vary from day to day, and sometimes from hour to hour. One may be operating at the need level for increased esteem, suddenly have an accident, and become overwhelmingly concerned with the physiological needs of being able to feed the family if one is incapacitated and unable to work. In spite of the limited applications of Maslow's theory, however, it does provide insight into the process of motivation and can often be useful in designing jobs, selecting staff, and developing strategies to maintain enthusiasm and interest among employees.

Frederick Herzberg, a contemporary of Maslow's, is credited with the "two-factor theory of motivation" or the "motivation-maintenance model," which complements Maslow's theory and provides additional perspectives.[8] Herzberg reviewed previous theories and studies and attempted to ascertain the essence of motivation by asking employees what they liked about their jobs and what they disliked about their jobs. After examining the data, he determined that the answers to the first question ("What do you like about your job?") were "motivation factors," while the answers to the second question ("What do you dislike about your job?") were what he termed "maintenance factors" (see Fig. 9-4). The five motivators he compiled in response to the first question were *the work itself*— being personally involved in the work, with a sense of responsibility and control; *achievement*—feeling personal accomplishment for having done a job well; *growth*—experiencing the opportunity for challenge in the job and the chance to learn skills and knowledge; *advancement*—knowing that the experience and growth will lead to increased responsibility and control; and *recognition*—being recognized for doing a job well, resulting in increased self-esteem.

Herzberg called the answers to the second question maintenance factors because he found that they maintained but did not improve current levels of production. Maintenance factors were *physical conditions*—e.g., lighting in the office and food in the cafeteria; *security*—a feeling of certainty about the future and of contentment; *economic factors*—salary and fringe benefits; and *social factors*— relationships with fellow workers and the boss.

Herzberg found that when the maintenance factors were poor, productivity decreased. Inadequate maintenance factors, then, hindered production, while adequate maintenance factors only maintained the current level. Thus, maintenance factors merely "satisfy" workers; they do not motivate them. As indicated in Figure 9-4, Herzberg's motivational factors are similar to those at the top of Maslow's "need priority" model, and his maintenance factors are toward the bottom of Maslow's model.

Motivation Through Enhancement of Self-Esteem. In the 1980s, particularly in the health professions, organizations have had to maintain as lean and as motivated a staff as possible to compete and to comply with governmental regulations. In the process of becoming "lean" by eliminating and combining as many positions as possible, those staff members who have survived may feel insecure, defensive, hostile, and fearful of losing their jobs, and may object to having had their former positions changed or enlarged without any monetary compensation. They may be unwilling to extend themselves because of the inference that the organization does not care about them. The manager or supervisor who is attempting to "motivate" staff under these conditions has a considerable challenge. While monetary increases are being kept to a minimum, the manager is expected to obtain more work from fewer people, who are already feeling unappreciated and overworked. Given this depressing but not unrealistic scenario, the manager needs to know and to exercise every motivational option available to him.

Many members of the current work force differ from their predecessors. Employees are more affluent and educated, and are less willing to rely on authority figures. They have different perceptions of themselves and are generally unwilling to tolerate a disrespectful supervisory style. What today's worker indicates he wants most is a heightened sense of self-esteem, realization, recognition, autonomy, responsibility, and a manager who recognizes his capacity for these achievements.[9] Although some employees can always be motivated by the hope of merit salary increases, the dietitian will benefit most from enhancing his staff's self-esteem and confidence as a prime method of increasing motivation to perform competently.

A great deal is known about the relationship between motivation and increased self-esteem or recognition. For more than half a century, social scientists have been aware of the phenomenon of the "self-fulfilling prophecy," which suggests that people perform and develop according to others' expectations of them. In one study, students and instructors were selected randomly, and some instructors were told that they had been selected to have all the brighter students in their classes. These instructors had students who performed statistically and significantly better than those in classes where instructors had no previous expectations.[10] Individuals who are told that they are incompetent and will be unable to achieve a specific goal or task perform poorly as compared with those who are told that they are competent and will be able to achieve the task, even though neither group has had previous experience with the task. An individual's self-perceived ability, based on previous performance, is positively related to later performance. Success begets success, and failure begets failure.[9]

Unfortunately, an appreciation of the implications of this phenomenon for business and industry has only recently become apparent. Whenever the supervisor acknowledges success in a subordinate, he adds to the likelihood that subsequent tasks will be performed successfully. For this reason, supervisors need to select carefully the right worker for the task, to provide adequate training to ensure employee success, and to assign work tasks that are manageable and accomplishable.

Dietitians can enhance the self-esteem of employees by providing opportunities for their achievement, growth, recognition, responsibility, and control, which increase their motivation to improve or to continue to do well. Several specific suggestions are described in the following paragraphs. They include involving employees in decision making, showing them respect, building their confidence, providing them with achievement experiences, increasing their personal and professional growth, and sharing time with them.

The dietitian must seek opportunities to observe and acknowledge his staff performing tasks properly. Employees are motivated when their esteem is enhanced through recognition of their work. The manner in which the work is recognized is a major factor in motivating employees. Simply saying "good job," for example, may be better than no comment at all, but it is not nearly as effective as a specific comment, such as, "the kitchen has never looked so organized. You did a splendid job of rearranging the storage cabinets." Needless to say, frequent reinforcement must be honest and must not sound patronizing.

Staff members can be motivated when they sense personal growth through their work. Learning new skills and exercising judgments can be motivating. When the dietitian believes a staff member is competent enough to succeed at a special assignment—one that is perceived as "job enrichment" and that offers an opportunity to develop skills—and he allows the employee adequate time to perform the new task successfully, he is, in fact, motivating him. Notice the qualifying comments in the preceding statement. A staff member should be selected only when the chances of success are high. Asking an employee to perform a task for which he is not prepared may decrease motivation. Adequate resources and time are critical to success.

Somewhat similar to the motivational effect of assigning special projects to staff is delegating responsibilities that had formerly been the supervisor's. When such assignments are made, it is important that they be given to employees who will not resent the added responsibility, but will see it as it is intended—as a form of recognition.

Taking the time to interact with employees on a person-to-person basis and listening to their comments about their work can be motivating when the employee perceives such interaction as a sign of respect and caring. The dietitian may be busy and prefer to go on working without acknowledging the employee; however, as being listened to is motivating, being ignored is non-motivating and demoralizing.

When employees make suggestions that the dietitian intends to consider, writing them down in the presence of the employee acknowledges that intention and decreases the possibility of the comments being forgotten. As with the other motivational strategies, however, the motivational potential of this technique will be short-lived if the employee interprets it as manipulation. When the dietitian writes down a suggestion, the expectation is that within a reasonable time, he will act on it. Accumulating and ignoring a drawer full of such suggestions will eventually discourage motivation in employees.

Acknowledging the feelings of employees who are obviously unhappy or excited is a way of showing caring and respect, as is recognizing important events in employees' lives. Attending funerals or sending flowers and greeting cards for specific occasions can be motivating if the employee perceives such acts as genuine signs of respect and recognition. Engaging in small talk with subordinates, visiting them for a few minutes, and asking about their families or commenting on new clothes all tend to go beyond the content of the message and express caring and acceptance of the employee.

Documenting some exceptional success provides the employee with a sense of recognition among the entire staff. For example, sending copies to the organization's director of a letter sent from a grateful client who comments on the work of an employee, and pinning a copy on the bulletin board, can provide recognition and build esteem.

If there is occasion to support the actions of subordinates and defend them to others in the organization, the dietitian should do so. All organizations have informal communication grapevines, and the employee will eventually hear that his supervisor extended himself on his behalf. Such actions have the potential to motivate many others as well, who, seeing themselves as members of the department's team, may vicariously feel defended as well.

The rationale for involving staff in decision making is discussed in detail in Chapter 6. When staff are consulted by their supervisor and involved in a decision, they not only tend to gain confidence from the experience, but also are motivated through the supervisor's appreciation of their worth.

Maintaining a motivated staff must be viewed as an ongoing process, and one that can be reinforced frequently through the quality of the dietitian's and employee's interaction. The dietitian's admitting when he is wrong, for example, and saying to a subordinate, "You are right," are actions that acknowledge respect for the subordinate. When problems arise in an employee's performance, the manner in which the assistance is offered or the employee is questioned is significant. Showing constructive concern in explaining the error adds to the employee's self-esteem; belittling, humiliating, or embarrassing an employee, especially in front of peers, diminishes it. Physical contact with subordinates can indicate caring and enhance self-esteem. Shaking hands with an employee or patting him on the back for a job well done are examples of human respect, caring, and affection, not sexual harassment. Many of the foregoing suggestions may seem obvious and simple, but it is their frequent absence that erodes the self-esteem of employees and inhibits their motivation to improve.

High turnover rates, mediocre performance, and chronic absenteeism are symptoms of the erosion of self-esteem and the inability of supervisors to develop it in staff. Several supervisors with whom one of the authors was working as a managerial consultant were asked whether they would be willing to make a special effort to give recognition, or a word of praise, to one of their workers for something he did well. Although they all claimed to be willing to do this, a subsequent meeting of the group found that none carried out the assignment. The reasons given included, "You just don't praise men," "Workers will think you are setting them up for something," and "It's a sign of weakness to praise people for what they do." One group member acknowledged that he simply did not know how to give praise.

Smiling and looking pleasant can also be a factor in maintaining a supportive relationship with staff. Employees cannot read the dietitian's mind, so if he looks angry and upset, the natural tendency is for the employee to infer that he, the employee, has somehow caused the unpleasant expression. A supervisor needs to monitor his nonverbal behavior so that it does not suggest negative messages unintentionally. When the supervisor is genuinely upset and subordinates are not at fault, they should be reassured that they are not the reason for his negative demeanor.

Providing employees with new equipment or other resource materials is another way to show confidence in their abilities, and it reinforces the impression that the dietitian wants them to succeed. Dietitians should try to learn from the employees themselves what they believe they need to work more efficiently. Whenever possible, employees should be provided with the resources requested.

A way to acknowledge excellence in a subordinate is to ask him to share his knowledge by teaching others. Giving the employee an assignment to train a new staff member, for example, is a form of recognition and a sign of confidence. Deferring to subordinates at meetings by asking them to explain procedures and solve problems accomplishes this as well.

Keeping and being on time for appointments with subordinates, notifying them well in advance if an appointment cannot be kept, and generally respecting the employee's time are signs of respect. Giving employees sufficient time to understand a particular procedure or set of directions, rather than leaving them feeling confused and insignificant, also adds to their perceptions of the supervisor's regard for them.

Motivation Through Setting Goals. Too often, subordinates believe that they are pleasing their supervisors only to learn that what they were doing was not what was desired or expected. When giving instructions, the dietitian should select language that is specific in meaning. Telling an employee to "work hard," to "be sincere," to "be confident," to "be conscientious," to "show cooperation," or to "maintain an open-minded point of view" are examples of vague instructions that could confuse an employee and cause him to fail. Telling an employee to "type a letter," "interview a patient," "conduct a performance appraisal," "investigate an accident," "ask questions," or "come to work on time" are examples of specific instructions that encourage success by allowing the employee to know exactly what is being asked of him.[9]

One of the most damaging on-the-job sources of stress is the absence or delay of feedback on one's performance.[9] Setting goals with subordinates as well as following up with subsequent periodic reviews provides feedback and promotes improved performance. Telling an employee, "Do your best," is useless. To the employee, who is faced with numerous alternatives for ways to spend his "working" time, this instruction can mean dozens of things. Setting goals complements the theories of Maslow and Herzberg. An effective way to assist others who wish to increase their esteem, growth, development, realization, and achievement is to teach them to be proactive in planning specific ways to accomplish more or to improve quality by setting goals.

The effect of setting goals on individual performance has been demonstrated. Theory and experiments support the proposition that supervisors should play an active role in setting goals with subordinates. Goals should be specific, clearly stated, and measurable. When they fulfill these conditions, they provide a criterion for feedback, accountability, and evaluation. An individual can be highly motivated by knowing the objective and working on a plan with the administrative dietitian to accomplish it. The three identifiable elements in goal setting are (1) an action verb, (2) a measurable result, and (3) the cost and/or date by which the objective will be accomplished. It is essential for both the employee and dietitian to agree on their mutual expectations, to clarify the difference, for example, between "I want you to get your work done soon," and "I want to see an increase of 10% by June 16th."

Individuals who have specific and challenging goals tend to perform best. Goals seen as "sure things" may discourage motivation as much as those that are believed to be impossible. The best goals— the ones that inspire quality performance—are those that are perceived as difficult and challenging but attainable. A major proposition, supported experimentally, is that employees who set or accept harder goals perform at levels superior to those who set or accept easier goals.[11]

Regardless of whether the goal is actually set by the dietitian or the employee, the two parties need to agree. When staff members feel that they are actively participating in setting their own goals, even if the goals are originally proposed by the supervisor, they are more solidly motivated to perform with distinction than if they feel that they are merely being told what to do. For the process to work, however, employees must trust their supervisors. When employees feel used, or when they feel that the goals are a means of exploiting them, they tend to resist the goals.

Motivation Through Reinforcement. Reinforcement, knowing how to encourage desirable behavior and to discourage undesirable behavior, is related to motivation. One way to increase the likelihood that a performance or behavior will recur is to follow the performance with a positive event. A positively reinforced response has a greater probability of recurring simply because it pays off. Most of the suggestions in the previous section on motivation through enhancement of self-esteem and recognition are examples of positive reinforcement.

Another type of reinforcement is the removal of something negative after the performance. In this case, the person is likely to repeat the behavior because something he dislikes is taken away as a consequence of the behavior. This removal or elimination of adverse conditions is referred to as negative reinforcement. A hospital dish washer, for example, who is constantly being checked by the dietitian and who has been able to decrease dish breakage by 30% from the previous month, will be motivated to continue improving if the dietitian checks this dish washer less often during the following week. The dietitian, then, can encourage the desired action by removing an unfavorable condition, the frequent inspections.

Two strategies that may discourage a given behavior are punishment and extinction. Reprimanding an employee for being late is an example of formal punishment. Although punishment is often used to eliminate undesireable behavior, its value is questionable because of its negative side effects. Punishment can make an employee hostile and prone to retaliation. If the punishment is perceived as unwarranted by the employee, he may resume the undesirable behavior as soon as punishment stops.

The other basic technique for decreasing the likelihood of a behavior is extinction. With extinction, the undesirable performance is neither punished nor rewarded; it is simply ignored. Ignored behaviors tend to diminish, and ultimately to become extinguished, as a result of a consistent lack of reinforcement. For example, a dietitian who never acknowledges an employee's suggestions is actually encouraging the employee to stop sending them. Although its use may be unintentional, extinction is an effective technique for terminating behavior. A manager should be aware of the potentially negative consequences of ignoring desired behavior. Motivated performances can be unintentionally extinguished by managers through carelessness.

Summary and Recommendations. Managers should give recognition to the employee in the presence of his peers. Recognition provides positive feedback and builds a worker's confidence and self-esteem. Organizations can benefit from involving their employees in the decision-making process. The more the employee is involved, the higher the level of his performance and satisfaction. Employees who participate in making decisions feel a sense of ownership and commitment.

Administrators at all levels lessen stress and increase efficiency and motivation when they provide employees with clearly defined goals and objectives. The more employees understand what they are expected to do, the more highly motivated they become. Supervisors should give respect and dignity to their staff. The more they respect the rights and privileges of the employee, the better the employee feels about himself and the more he produces. Managers must become familiar with reinforcement techniques, training themselves to recognize and comment on good work in order to reinforce it. Ignoring good work may lead to extinction of desired behavior. Top management needs to instill in lower-level management an appreciation of the human resources of the organization, supporting the development of increased self-esteem, recognition, and growth among all staff.

This chapter has emphasized the complexity of motivation and has discussed its behavioral implications for dietitians. Dietitians are involved daily with motivation of both staff and clients. Understanding motivational concepts and being able to employ the strategies and techniques associated with them can add immeasurably to the professional's effectiveness.

SUGGESTED ACTIVITIES

1. List the factors that motivate you to go to work or to continue with your present job. Explain your reactions in terms of the Maslow and Herzberg models.

2. Interview someone who is on a diet, and determine the positive and negative influences for motivation that have resulted from adherence to it. Discuss your interview and data using the variables motivating change in food choices and health behavior model presented in the chapter (see Fig. 9-1).

3. Examine the forces that motivate you to learn something new. Are they related to your desire to remain physically well, secure, well-liked and respected, or are they related to your desire to prepare yourself for taking on additional responsibility, having more control, and achieving realization and actualization?

4. Indicate why the following statements would have a negative impact on an employee's motivation and how they might be amended so that they maintain the employee's self-esteem.

A. That job has been done incorrectly! What do I have to do to get you to understand?

B. I'm tired of listening to you complain. Just keep still and do your job.

C. You will probably make a mess of this, but there isn't anyone else to do it.

D. If you would listen, you would understand.

E. You can't be serious about that suggestion.

5. For each of the following examples, list the reinforcement technique used and the feelings it might produce in the employee.

A. Employee: Mrs. Jones, since you told us to be on the lookout for problems with equipment, we have discovered two more.

Dietitian: Yes, but I'm looking for Helen now. Have you seen her?

B. Employee: Mrs. Jones, I've finished all the work in the kitchen and have begun to rearrange the cabinets.

Dietitian: You mean it took you all this time just to do that?

C. Dietitian: Mary, I am putting you on suspension for three days.

D. Dietitian: Mary, I want you to know that I appreciate how effectively you work with others. Several people have told me how thorough you are in using the new procedures.

Answers:

5A. Extinction. The employee would probably feel ignored and rejected.

5B. Punishment. The employee would probably feel angry and defensive.

5C. Punishment. The employee's feelings would be affected by whether she felt that the punishment was warranted. If she felt it was unwarranted, she would feel angry.

5D. Positive reinforcement. The employee would probably feel appreciated and respected.

REFERENCES

1. Wlodkowski, R.J.: Motivation and Teaching. Washington, DC, National Education Assoc., 1984.
2. Peckos, P.S.: Stimulating the patient in self-motivation. J. Am. Diet. Assoc., *61*:423, 1972.
3. Krondl, M., and Lau, D.: Social determinants in human food selection. *In* The Psychobiology of Human Food Selection. Edited by L.M. Baker. Westport, CT, AVI Publishing Co., 1982.
4. Hochbaum, G.M.: Behavior and education. *In* Nutrition, Lipids, and Coronary Heart Disease. Edited by R. Levy et al. New York, Raven Press, 1979.
5. Hochbaum, G.M.: Strategies and their rationale for changing people's eating habits. J. Nutr. Ed., *13*:S59, 1981.
6. Johnson, D.W., and Johnson, R.T.: Nutrition education's theoretical foundation. J. Nutr. Ed. *17*:S8, 1985.
7. Maslow, A.H.: Motivation and Personality. New York, Harper and Bros., 1954.
8. Herzberg, F.: Work and the Nature of Man. Cleveland, World Publishing Co., 1966.
9. Rosenbaum, B.L.: How To Motivate Today's Workers. New York, McGraw-Hill, 1982.
10. Rosenthal, R., and Jacobson, L.: Pygmalion in the Classroom. New York, Rinehart and Winston, 1968.
11. Chruden, H.J., and Sherman, A.W., Jr.: Managing Human Resources. 7th ed. Cincinnati, South-Western Publishing Co., 1984.

Appendices

APPENDIX A

Diet History Form

NAME _____ Age, height, weight _____

Current diet _____

Breakfast (time and place):

Food Frequency
(amount per day/week):

Milk, dairy
Coffee, tea
Alcohol
Other beverages
Fruit, juice
Vegetables
Lunch (time and place):   Bread/cereal
Meat, poultry, fish
Eggs
Fats and oils
Sweets

Dinner (time and place):

Snacks (time and place):

Antecedents (cues to eating):

Eating behaviors:

Eating consequences
(reinforcement):

APPENDIX B

Counseling Guidelines—Initial Session

Step	Topic	Questions to Ask	Questions to Avoid
1.	*Candidly review the problems of dietary change.*		
	1. Review overall rationale and objectives for recommended diet.		
	2. Acknowledge difficult nature of dietary change.	What are your thoughts and feelings about this diet?	Do you have any opinion about this diet?
	3. Listen to patient's concerns about the recommended diet.		
2.	*Build some commitment to solve problems.*		
	1. Indicate your willingness to work with patient.		
	2. Clarify to patient that he must assume primary responsibility for making dietary changes.		
	3. Propose program of frequent meetings over next 3 months, close self-observation of diet, phone contact.		
	4. *Emphasize* slow but steady approach to change.		
	5. Obtain patient's verbal commitment to meet any of your proposals.	What aspects of this program are you willing to try now?	Do you want to try anything now?

Counseling Guidelines—Initial Session (Continued)

Step	Topic	Questions to Ask	Questions to Avoid
3.	*Plan some specific changes in diet during coming month.*		
	1. Emphasize good points of 3-day record.*		
	2. Look on record for ideas on dietary changes.		
	3. Probe patient for more ideas.		
	4. Pinpoint *one* aspect of diet pattern to change.	What do you see that could be changed or improved?	Do you see anything to change?
	5. Acknowledge patient's desire for radical and fast changes in diet, but re-emphasize that the most successful approach is slow and steady.		
	6. Help patient set realistic dietary change goals (e.g., one meatless evening meal per week, substitution of a salad bowl for usual main entree at one lunch per week).	What is a realistic goal for you?	Is this a realistic goal?
4.	*Plan how to make a change successful.*		
	1. Identify problems that are likely to interfere with achieving goal. Consider problems in the following areas:	What problems are likely to interfere with your plans?	Are any problems going to interfere with your plans?
	a. *Physical environment* (e.g., what foods are available in house, snacking in front of T.V. in evening, absence of reminders on refrigerator or dining table)	What can you change in your home, office, or car that will help you achieve your goal?	Do you need any reminders?
	b. *Social environment* (e.g., influential people, such as spouse, children, business associates, whose approval and support—criticism—can affect achievement of dietary change goal)	Who can help, what can they do, and what can I do to help during the next few weeks?	Do you need any help?

* Prior to initial counseling session, patient should be given materials and instructions for completing a 3-day food diary.

Counseling Guidelines—Initial Session (Continued)

Step	Topic	Questions to Ask	Questions to Avoid
	c. *Cognitive or private environment* (e.g., what patient says to himself when confronted with personal thoughts such as the following) —what others will say about his planned behavior —thoughts of failure or disappointment when he is not perfect in his behavior	What encouraging things can you say to yourself when confronted with these inevitable thoughts?	Will you give yourself encouragement?
5.	*Plan how to keep track of progress.* Devise an unobtrusive and convenient way for patient to keep a record of the desired or target behavior (e.g., count egg cartons, measure side of vegetable oil container, attach pencil *and* paper to refrigerator, table, wallet, etc.)	How are you going to keep track of (target behavior)?	Can you keep track of (target behavior)?
6.	*Plan counseling continuity and support.*	When is it convenient for me to call and discuss your progress? When can we schedule our next appointment?	Do you want me to contact you sometime?
7.	*Make certain that spouse, if present, is involved in answering questions, providing ideas, and discussing potential problems and solutions.*		

From Wilbur, C.S.: Nutrition Counseling Skills. Audio Cassette Series 5. Chicago, The American Dietetic Association, 1980.

APPENDIX C

Counseling Guidelines—Follow-Up Sessions

Step	Topic	Questions to Ask	Questions to Avoid
1.	*Review patient's progress.* Emphasize the positive and check commitment.*	What thoughts do you have about this approach to lowering your cholesterol?	Do you have any thoughts about this approach to counseling?
2.	*Discuss the problems that interfered with achieving the goal and how patient attempted to solve them.*	What problems did you face?	Did you have any problems?
3.	*Plan next specific change in diet for coming month.*		
	a. Look at old food record for ideas.		
	b. Probe patient for ideas.	What do you see that could be changed or improved?	Do you see anything to change?
	c. Pinpoint *one* aspect of diet pattern to change.		
	d. Reacknowledge patient's probable desire to make fast, radical changes, but re-emphasize the importance of slow but steady approach.		
	e. Set a realistic behavior change goal.		
	f. *Include plans for patient to continue with the changes he accomplished last month.*		
4.	*Plan how to make change successful.*		
	1. Identify problems that are likely to interfere with achieving goal. Consider problems in the following areas a through c.	What problems are likely to interfere with your plans?	Are any problems going to interfere with your plans?

* Be prepared to handle *either* the patient's success *or* failure in achieving previous goal.

Counseling Guidelines—Follow-Up Sessions (Continued)

Step	Topic	Questions to Ask	Questions to Avoid
	a. *Physical environment* (e.g., what foods are available in house, snacking in front of T.V. in evening, absence of reminders on refrigerator or dining table)	What can you change in your home, office, or car that will help you achieve your goal?	Do you need any reminders?
	b. *Social environment* (e.g., influential people, such as spouse, children, business associates, whose approval and support—or criticism—can affect achievement of dietary change goal)	Who can help, what can they do, and what can I do to help during the next few weeks?	Do you need any help?
	c. *Cognitive or private environment* (e.g., what patient says to himself when confronted with personal thoughts such as the following:	What encouraging things can you say to yourself when confronted with these inevitable thoughts?	Will you give yourself encouragement?
	—What others will say about his planned behavior	Other's approval	
	—Thoughts of failure or disappointment when he is not perfect in his behavior		
	—Negative feelings (hunger, irritability) that *will* accompany behavior change	Negative reactions to change	
	—Feeling goal not as important as once thought (usually 4–5 days after counseling session)	Devaluation of goal over time	
5.	*Plan how to keep track of progress.*		
	Devise an unobtrusive and convenient way for patient to keep a record of the desired or target behavior (e.g., count egg cartons, measure side of vegetable oil container, attach pencil *and* paper to refrigerator, table, wallet, etc.)	How are you going to keep track of (target behavior)?	Can you keep track of (target behavior)?

Counseling Guidelines—Follow-Up Sessions (Continued)

Step	Topic	Questions to Ask	Questions to Avoid
6.	*Plan counseling continuity and support.*	When is it convenient for me to call and discuss your progress? When can we schedule our next appointment?	Do you want me to contact you sometime?
7.	*Make certain that spouse, if present, is involved in answering questions, providing ideas, discussing potential problems and solutions.*		

From Wilbur, C.S.: Nutrition Counseling Skills. Audio Cassette Series 5. Chicago, The American Dietetic Association, 1980.

APPENDIX D

Interview Evaluation Form

Parts of the Interview	Quality	Suggestions for Improvement
Preplanning Interview guide		
Physical environment		
Patient context		
Psychologic privacy		
Opening Greeting		
Statement of purpose		
Development of rapport		
Physical comfort		
Nonverbal signals		
Interviewer		
Respondent		
Body of Interview Sequence of topics		
Maintenance of rapport		
Nonverbal signals		
Interviewer		
Respondent		
Questions Open-ended		
Closed		
Primary		
Secondary		
Leading		
Neutral		
Probes		
Clarification		
Paraphrase		
Repetition		
Summary		

Interview Evaluation Form (Continued)

Parts of the Interview	Quality	Suggestions for Improvement
Use of silence		
Responses Understanding		
Confrontational		
Evaluative		
Hostile		
Reassuring		
Pace of interview		
Vocabulary level		
Talking vs. listening (%)		
Closing Appreciation		
Questions requested		
Future contacts		
Nonverbal signals		
Interviewer		
Respondent		

Note: A numerical scale such as very good (3), adequate (2), and needs improvement (1) may be used. A tally system may be used to count the different kinds of questions asked.

INDEX

Page numbers in *italics* indicate figures.